"Juggling Manure"

Living With Cancer

LESLEY WHITEHEAD

"Juggling Manure"

Living With Cancer

Matador
9 De Montfort Mews
Leicester LE1 7FW, UK
Tel: (+44) 116 255 9311 / 9312
Email: books@troubador.co.uk
Web: www.troubador.co.uk/matador

ISBN 978-1905886-494

Every effort has been made to trace the copyright holders of material quoted in
this book. However, should any have been omitted, the Author will be pleased to make
full acknowledgement in future editions.

Wild Goose Worship Group
From "A Wee Worship Book" © 1999, WGRG, Iona Community, G2 3DH.

Typeset in 11pt Stempel Garamond by Troubador Publishing Ltd, Leicester, UK
Printed in the UK by The Cromwell Press Ltd, Trowbridge, Wilts, UK

Matador is an imprint of Troubador Publishing Ltd

"I am absolutely not a victim...if my mother had been alive, she would have said, 'It's jolly bad luck, old girl. You have to deal with it as best you can.' And that's exactly what I'm doing."
[Polly Havers of her battle with ovarian cancer]

"I've learned to embrace it, but I don't want it to define me."
[Christopher Reeve "Superman" of his disability]

"Never juggle manure."
[Clive's Cat's Cartoons]

"Creative Courage, then, is the Quintessential ingredient in Elemental Feminist Genius. It moves/stirs creating Crones to Realize in the material world the forms/Exemplars that are taking shape in our minds...

Our Radical Elemental Feminist creations are specific to us as individuals. For one at one time it may be a book...

As Concreators we work in harmony. At times this harmony/accord is conscious. Sometimes it is subliminally sensed."
[Daly 1998 : 97]

PROLOGUE: 6 DECEMBER 1996

★

A date forever imprinted on my memory. The day when I first discovered what it is like to go into shock, when my consultant surgeon called me back into hospital to tell me that the results of a recent biopsy showed simultaneous breast cancers, which had both spread into my lymph system.

To be honest, the shock of that consultation and the rapid onset of the cancer treatment that followed meant that (at that time) I didn't fully take on board the implications of the diagnosis that had just been delivered to me. Maybe that was a good thing – knowing what I know now about the disease with which I live, I don't imagine that any of the nursing staff who first dealt with my case expected me still to be around the magic five years after initial diagnosis. Yet, over eight years later, thanks to the time and place in which I live, I'm still here...

Part One

September 2001 – April 2002

"…she looked again at the azalea and noted what unusually large single blossoms it had, and she felt that this looking, this still intense joy in a flower, was her way of praising God."

[May Sarton]

JOURNAL, 4 SEPTEMBER 2001

★

Travelling down to the south coast on Friday (for James' welcome service in his new church), I was conscious of the last few hours of officially being a Superintendent Minister. I was somewhat surprised (though I have always felt that I had made the right decision in withdrawing from this position of responsibility), to discover the feeling of relief that was within me, when Saturday 1st September dawned, and I no longer held that position, even in name. For all practical purposes I ceased doing the job when my sick leave began in April, but having already set up all necessary cover for the ensuing period, it is only at this late stage that I feel my responsibilities in the role have really ended and I am feeling daily more relieved about the change.

It is similar to the unexpected relief I felt when Jeremy and Katie flew off to Greece in July, whilst Jamie was on exchange in Germany. Going to the airport with Dad, I had been anxious about their journey. As they passed through the departure doors, I felt nothing but a lifting of responsibility and relief. I conclude that I have had too much responsibility for too long and need a period to sit back and recover; and take more responsibility for my own well-being.

What does feel strange is to enter into a New Year as far as Methodism is concerned (the eleventh of my ministry within the Methodist Church) and to be on sick leave. It is the first time that

I have not been working at the start of the New Year. However, if things only progress as they are doing (i.e. if I manage to get back to work after just six months off), by the end of this year, I will have had nine months off in total (I had three after my mastectomy in 1997). Does nine months out of eleven years sound a lot? Even though it's not my fault that I have had cancer at all, that particular statistic makes me sound a liability to employers. Even though I know I have probably done the job of several people whenever I have been working (and people seem to recognize that by asking me to stay longer here and saying I must take as long as I need to get well again), that is a hard statistic to swallow. There is a sense of failure about it that can be hard to reconcile.

I think that I have worked too hard for too long. Is cancer the result of that, I sometimes wonder? It's certainly not much of a reward for trying so hard for so long. But alongside my cancer has come a kind of gift – that of time to be myself, whoever that might be, though, in a sense, that time is still to be discovered. For the first part of my time off, I was just coping physically with getting from day to day. Then came the school holidays and demands for time and attention from the children (albeit very different demands from when they were little). Today was our first day without them...and even then the demands were till the very last minute of their leaving for school, despite the fact that I had tried hard to have everything ready on time.

JOURNAL,
THURSDAY 13 SEPTEMBER 2001

★

I still find it hard to believe the way in which time passes, when I am apparently doing nothing in particular with it. I have now been on sick leave for five months and so much has changed in terms of who I am and my circumstances, all because of what felt like a pea-sized lump in the nape of my neck, though I was later told that it was bigger than that. Would an inventory be helpful or hurtful? Let's try and see. I anticipate this will be a painful exercise, in terms of feelings of loss and grief, which are already beginning as I contemplate the situation.

(i) After ten years of full-time ministry, I had carefully set up my sabbatical of three months, which I felt that I deserved and to which I was looking forward. I was going to spend a month in Texas – part study, part travelling and was going to see Jose (on Death Row) in the process. My acquaintance with Texas began through Jose four years ago. I was looking forward to the time that I would be able to spend with Jamie as my travelling companion and I feel like I have been cheated of that time with him. Besides, I still haven't had that holiday abroad with Mum and Dad, which is maybe why I am hesitant of booking up to go to Madeira with them at the end of October – feels like tempting fate. These feelings are made more intense, because Jamie is growing up so fast and time to be with him is running out – he will have his own life to lead. And I have strong feelings about spending time with Mum and Dad while we can, because they are growing noticeably older, and my feelings about their mortality are heightened, as I have to cope with my own.

(ii) In the process, I have had to step aside from my MA. Instead of being able to use my sabbatical to crack on with it, I have had to drop ideas of studying in Perkins Seminary in Dallas, of having time at Queens' College, Birmingham and of graduating from Oxford with a Master of Theology in October 2002. My brain has turned to jelly and concentration and language are difficult, partly due to stress and partly to the well-documented side effects of menopause, into which I have been plunged. At this stage in writing (what, three paragraphs since beginning?), I am exhausted with the effort of what I have so far managed. Me, the person who took on an MA to get away from thinking of cancer (ironic?), who gradually brought an addled brain round after a bilateral mastectomy to being able to write essays (which had seemed unbelievable at the start) of 3, 4 or 5,000 words. Now after three paragraphs, I struggle to continue.

(iii) In five months I have gone from suspecting that being on Tamoxifen for four and a half years was beginning to start me on the menopausal route (periods less regular and very heavy when they came) to being plunged startlingly into menopause head-first and trying to come to terms with its side effects, as opposed to the side effects of my hormonal medication, or even my anti-depressants. The route has been via two operations under general anaesthetic. The first was in April, which involved seeing my surgeon on Maundy Thursday and being told (despite an Easter Bank Holiday weekend intervening), "come into hospital next Tuesday and I'll operate on Wednesday". The second (even more stunning) was in June, seeing a gynaecologist who specializes in cancer on a Monday, to be told (after lengthy discussion about what I wanted to happen), "come into hospital tomorrow and I'll do you a complete hysterectomy on Wednesday". I must confess that the fact that everyone reckons he is a very dishy doctor completely passed me by on that occasion!

(iv) I started off five months ago breastless. Now I am womb and ovary less as well. I have had two bilateral operations – bilateral mastectomy and bilateral oophorectomy (ovaries) included with my hysterctomy. But then, I started off with simultaneous bloody cancers, so I obviously don't do anything by halves!

I can't do any more itemizing. It is too painful to list all that has been lost in the last five months (including my ability to work, my position as a Superintendent Minister, my ability to have any more children ever). I have run out of energy and inclination, though overall, in the last few days, I have to say that I am beginning to feel better in myself than I have for quite a while. (If we ignore the world situation pre-empted by the terrorist acts in the States, that is.)

Talking about the cancers and ops, as in (iv) above serves to underline the fact that I probably (statistically) shouldn't be here at all; and reminds me that I have no guarantees about being here in the future. But then I have to stick with John Diamond's assessment of statistics (50/50), and say, "hey, I'll either make it or I won't and so far, look on the good side, and see that you've made it this far when the odds were stacked against you".

It takes a lot of energy to remain positive. I know my oncologist was surprised at the speed at which my tumour shrank with the Arimidex, just like the previous oncologist (now retired) was surprised and pleased at how well my previous tumours responded to chemotherapy. And I know without a doubt that the prayers and support of community is key in coming through such difficult circumstances; but nevertheless, there are times when it is hard. Like when my friend rings to tell me she's home from hospital after her bone marrow transplant; and I am genuinely pleased for her, when she says that her doctors have said that if she carries on as she is, in three months time they will be able to start talking in terms of cure. The odds she has come through to get here are amazing and I am pleased for her. The only 'but' comes in terms of knowing that no-one is likely to be talking in terms of cure for me; because they won't do that with breast cancer – it's too unpredictable. I could be clear for the next twenty years and then it might turn up unexpectedly in my bones or liver or even, God forbid, my head.

Then, in terms of identity – who am I, and who do other people think I am? Sometimes I am intrigued to read cards people send me, because I wonder who or what they are talking about. For instance, a friend from Methodism writes to wish me well and "hope you are progressing after your set back". What is being said of me in public? Is my cancer recurrence seen as a setback in my recovery since the first lot? I had a long remission (over four years) from the first time. This is a new development. If it was the first lot still, I'd have been long dead by now. Don't mistake me, I value the love and good wishes of people, who are only trying their best to find words in a difficult and maybe for them unimaginable situation, but I just wonder who they mean in their writing. Is it me?

Then again, I had a supportive letter from the Secretary of the Methodist District today, which included the words, "we are inspired by the courage and determination you have shown........." Whilst it is lovely to have such words directed in my direction, I go along with John Diamond again, and question that what I am showing is courage. There seems to be a choice – either get on with it or don't; but as that is as far as the choice goes and what makes you courageous or determined just because you opt to get on with it? If you had real choice, you wouldn't battle on, you'd step out of the circumstances and leave the bravery to someone else, thanks very much. Bravery is not my choice – a cancer-free life might be (i.e. never to have had it in the first place).

The preacher in a sermon last week said he felt that he might metaphorically jump out of the aeroplane if he was in a situation of danger, rather than going on to face the danger. I said to him, what if you can't jump out of the aeroplane? I can't choose to jump out of my cancer. I'm in my body and stuck with it. How can I be brave, when I don't even have the choice to step aside from the danger? It's not brave to not even consider suicide, when life is what you want so badly. In retrospect, his illustration was highly ironic anyway; as the Americans on those hijacked planes had no choice to jump either. And there I will stop, because the consequences of what has happened in the States this week, could far outweigh the significance of me as an individual struggling with cancer. We could be looking at the possibility of a third world war, unless considered action is taking in response to this terrorism. But that's a-whole-nother subject, way beyond the remit of this journal.

EMAIL OF WEEK BEGINNING
17 SEPTEMBER 2001

*

Hi Chris – Ethel brought me a couple of the posters you did for distribution re current anxiety-making world situation. Thank you for those. Everyone seems to be singing your praises! Which just goes to prove what I have always suspected – that we are none of us indispensable, and by the time I'm fully fit again, there won't be a job for me to come back to hereabouts! I imagine the grapevine has told you, however, that if anyone can find a way for me to make a few pennies to rub together, the churches have invited me to stay two more years after this one – till August 2004, in fact. Can you stand the stress?

Maybe one day I will be able to make coherent conversation again, and not have people groping for possible words to help me out of a sticky situation. And maybe there may again come a day when I can be up, dressed and breakfasted somewhere before 10.30 or 11am. Hey ho! It is a very salutary experience, when someone who has recently been capable of studying for a Diploma through Oxford University, is no longer able to keep concentrating beyond two paragraphs of a journal for her counsellor, or for more than two emails or one letter at a time.

Today I have made a casserole in the slow cooker, baked a bread and butter pudding (for the first time ever) and fetched Katie from school (via the tram, as my car was in for MOT). I took the children to the dentist (five minutes walk) and that is the sum of my achievements. Today I even felt too paltry to hang out the washing or wash the lunch dishes, both of which tasks Ethel magnanimously undertook, having first of all hoovered and dusted the entire house from top to bottom, and cleaned all kitchen, bathroom and toilet floors as well. Ethel is seventy and I used to do the bits I mentioned at top speed around a day's work (apart from the never-before-baked bread and butter pudding). I don't think I will ever be able to adequately express to someone who hasn't been in the situation how this all makes me feel. The only compensation is that I hope (intend) to get better gradually and that I hope I am not going to sink further into mental oblivion, as someone like my friend with dementia seems likely to do. In fact, I may not die for a while yet, but then again, who knows?! And then what about all the people who were struggling with cancer, families, bereavement, all the usual ★★★★★★ bits of life when some bloody idiots blew them to bits (literally) by crashing ★★★★★★★ aeroplanes into their places of work last week? Some days I feel about one hundred and fifty.

The things that keep me sane are my rabbit (who has got a wonderful winter coat and new mane – she's a Lionhead), Katie's guinea pigs, the cats, and the children, I think. Though it was not easy having to explain to Jamie today why it is a BIT OF A WORRY that Pakistan has nuclear missiles trained on India. "What's that got to do with collapsing world trade centres Mum?"

Jeremy also keeps me sane. I didn't forget. I just take him for granted. Or I did. I don't think I can take things or people for granted any more. I hope the aged parent is coping with Jacob and Sophie? And I hope that Sarah is never taken for granted in all your comings and goings!

"My God", he says, "I wish I'd never met this woman!" Sorry, this email, like Topsy, just growed! I think I may add a bit of it to my journal. Because there were occasions when I wrote, when I felt VERY angry. Guess which bits! My counsellor thinks I need to use the space with her just to feel all these things. She's actually very good and interactive. She will help a lot, I think.

All the Best, from Lesley.

HOLIDAY REFLECTIONS AND
READING REVISITED

★

Every life has its way markers. For me, the journey through the landscape of cancer has been managed with the help of key people, some of whom I have only met in the pages of a book. For instance, I wonder if I could have survived thus far, if I had not "met" with John Diamond (1999) when I read "C: Because Cowards Get Cancer Too"? Incidentally, I believe very strongly that this book should be obligatory reading for any person dealing with cancer on a professional level – to show that we, the cancer patients, are people too, though we may be struggling with our identity as such:

> "...the fact remained: I was not me any more. That my friends seemed to be willing to do almost anything for me was, I believed in those mad moments, almost worse: they were responding to who I was before the operation rather than who I had become after it...
> ...this is what disease does to us. It wrecks our faces and our voices and any talents we may have lying around, and then it makes us desperately depressed so that we're unable to deal with the wreckage."
> (p.170)

I would add that, it might also depress our partners, so that they too experience some difficulty in dealing with life. Then again:

> "... I felt the oppressive weight of the interminable surgical process suddenly, slicing me inch-by-inch, suckering me into ever more drastic remedies, ever more unbearable disabilities..." (p.249)

Meditating on John Diamond and all the physical traumas inflicted on him, not by the cancer itself, but in order to cure the cancer, or give him a longer span of life, than he would otherwise have had, I realise (perhaps for the first time) the enormous physical changes that have been wrought upon my body for the same reasons. I have always just kind of taken for granted my "collection of scars", but actually they need to be seen in terms of physical changes that have come about in order to monitor and curb cancer.

Cancer was the motivation behind the two big surgeries I have had – the two bilaterals. I feel very down when I think that – as it puts me very clearly in the league of "cancer patient". Which maybe I have always denied (refused to see myself as). The question is – do I lessen my lifespan by becoming that (i.e. a cancer patient)? Does it make death more inevitable than denying the diagnosis seems to do? In other words, is it safe to look at what it means to be a "cancer patient"? Can I come out the other side of that recognition? Or is such a fear the reason why I am really quite reluctant to bury a friend's ashes (who died of cancer) in a position of daily view?

JOURNAL,
THURSDAY 20 SEPTEMBER 2001

★

Have just been re-reading my journal so far and there are several things I need to pick up on.

"Time to be myself..." I think that I am literally only just, in these last two days, beginning to have any time by myself to reflect on all that has happened recently. Yesterday I opted out of a lunch engagement with Jeremy and our friend, because I was so tired. I couldn't get up and when I did get up, I just sat and had quiet time and wrote a few thank you notes (at last) to people who have sent me cards and good wishes over these last months. I had a sandwich and then watched afternoon TV until it was time to get Katie from school..........then all the "jobs" began again. I can't believe how exhausted I am. I think I must be depressed, or maybe it's just trying to take the time and look at what has happened. I also feel sick. Bodies continue to amaze me – both with their ability to heal themselves and their ability to produce physical symptoms like exhaustion and sickness to tell you there is something mentally/emotionally/spiritually wrong.

"It takes a lot of energy to remain positive." That's the other way of seeing days like yesterday and today. Because most of the time I try to be positive in getting up, washed, dressed, exercising, etc, I forget how much energy this uses up in a recovering body. So

every now and then said body refuses to cooperate, whilst taking a chance to get its breath back.

"If you had real choice, you wouldn't battle on, you'd... leave the bravery to someone else, thanks very much." Every now and then, I feel like saying to someone, "O.K. The game's over now. I've played the part long enough. Can we go back to how things were please? Can you return me to my reality?" The trouble is, I don't know what my reality is any more and that is very scary.

"I'm in my body and stuck with it." The sheer physicality of what has happened to me sometimes overwhelms me. It affects my ability to walk any distance, or makes me very tired in retrospect the next day if I do any exercise. If I don't exercise, my joints all stiffen up and I waddle like a penguin. Even now, I daren't pull or push anything heavy. If I even so much as try it, I end up with pain in my stomach. Aches and pains all over, but especially under my left arm scare me to death. Who do I tell those fears to?

So the litany begins....
"The lump has gone in your neck" (check to affirm, note tenderness there). "Therefore, if there were cancer anywhere else, it would have been similarly affected by Arimidex."
"Yes, but what if it were starting again?"
"I know the Arimidex may stop being effective at some stage, but it won't be yet"
"What about that cough?"
"You've only had it since the anaesthetic, and anyway your chest X-ray was clear."

It's no wonder I end up feeling exhausted. The energy required to stay on top of all this is immense. That's without the hot sweats, which are just overwhelming at times. A friend told me she used to just imagine a cool wind, until she cooled down. I can't do that. Every time I try, I know that I just have to get as many of my clothes off as possible and get out in the air if I can. Am I going to be sitting with the back door open in the winter in my underwear, whilst the rest of the family shiver in their woolies?

"The Americans on those hijacked planes had no choice to jump either." But the people who jumped from the World Trade Towers had choice. In a lose-lose situation, I think it was perhaps very brave to hurl yourself to certain death, rather than wait till the smoke and flames got you.

"The consequences of what has happened in the States this week, could far outweigh the significance of me as an individual struggling with cancer" The grief has somehow been intertwined over recent days, of the struggle to cope with my own situation and the consequences of the terrorist activity. The huge humanitarian crisis unfolding over Afghanistan's borders – people who don't even have the basic necessities of life like food, let alone medical aid. Millions of people who die without hope of a better kind of life. And here's me, knowing that I can't survive without the best medicine that the West has to offer me. If my medication were cut off by war, I would be in at least as much danger as anyone on the battle front. Why do the 'I' and 'me' loom so large? Is it because it is all we can know or be sure of? The ego has to be big to survive?

"Living with cancer must always mean living with the threat of death…"(Diamond, 1999 : 255)
A lot of the above shows, I think, that I am finding it hard to wrestle with the idea of my own mortality. That struggle is

enhanced/more clearly defined by huge events that show the fragility of mortality for everyone. If I could sit more lightly to all this, maybe I would be able to find a way through it? But I am terrified of dying, because of leaving those I love to cope without my support.

EMAIL TO IAN, 9 OCTOBER 2001

★

I am starting a course of antibiotics. I have had a lovely "girls' only" weekend near Whitby. Weather was bright and autumnal. I had a heavy cold though, which has ended with the gland under my chin swelling. Consulted with my GP and my oncologist's secretary today. I think (and Dr M. agrees) that it's an infection. Dr C. says (via secretary) that if it doesn't settle down with antibiotics, I should ring and he'll see me again. My next appointment with him is on November 7 anyway, so I should be OK till then. I don't think it's cancer, but this whole round of everything can be so wearying. In with everything else, I've also got some eczema on my right arm now. Grrrrr!! Anyway, whatever happens I am going to go on planned holiday to Madeira with my parents on October 29th (precluding outbreak of World War Three, of course).

It is the cancer that it is hardest to get your head round as you recover. Also, the lack of time to myself. Today has been taken up with illness. Now just when I thought it OK to have some time to myself, someone wants me again. Sometimes I don't feel like I have time to think or be. I just cope with each thing as it comes up, whether it is a physical problem of mine, or a problem with one of the children, or the animals...

I cannot believe that six months off work have passed. I feel like I've done nothing, and yet I am beginning to think of having to go back. I need an aim, so I'm considering starting off gently in December. I asked for another sick note today. The Dr said, did I want another three months, but we've gone for eight weeks for now. I will go back and get another note if I can't manage to start work again then. I didn't intend to offload all this on you. I decided against doing any of my journal tonight (for my counsellor), because I knew I wouldn't have much "free" time. I can't believe how angry I feel about not having any space to think about what is happening to me. I expect I will cut an excerpt of this email and paste it in my journal...

JOURNAL,
THURSDAY 11 OCTOBER 2001

★

"Living with cancer must always mean living with the threat of death even, I imagine, if you manage to increase the distance between you and the diagnosis to the five years which counts as a cure." (Diamond, 1999 : 255)

I have come to the conclusion after our weekend away and conversations with various friends, that the thing I really have to try and face up to this time round is my own death – the likelihood of it, the possibility of it. I feel that I never really grasped that the last time I had cancer – that I found it unbelievable even.

"My guess is that the first time you can accept the possibility of a cure and arrange your terror to fit in with the medical optimism. A second time and you're there on your own." (Diamond, 1999 : 230)

Interestingly though, Jeremy (in conversation at lunch today) admitted that he had seen it as a possibility last time. But then I keep finding out things that he thought of, or was aware of, in the context of my illness and treatment, that he knew and never told me, because he thought they weren't helpful for me at the time. So when I discover something and say "Did you know?" he says, "Yes, I knew that". How did he bear to keep such painful things to himself? He has often been very strong for me. Have I appreciated it? He kind of works the gradual disclosure principal of the doctors; they always answer your questions, though they never tell you more than you ask and, I guess, that I only ask what I need to know at any given time.

Previously in this journal, I have asked myself, "Do I lessen my lifespan by becoming...a 'cancer patient'? Does it make death more inevitable than denying the diagnosis seems to do?" Now, I really feel that, I have to tackle the idea of my own dying. I have some sense that if I could do this successfully – give up clinging to life, if you like, I would be able to live more comfortably in however many years are left to me on this planet. If I were to live another forty years, I can't spend them all being afraid of dying. And if my life span is to be shorter than that, I want to enjoy it, not spend all my time being afraid. There is the tension between the sentiment echoed in the Travis song and the words of Dylan Thomas. Travis (2001) sing:

> "Well I believe there's someone watching over you
> They're watching every single thing you say
> And when you die they'll set you down and take you through...."
> ("Side" from the album "The Invisible band")

Whereas, Dylan Thomas shouts fiercely, "Do not go gentle into that good night" and continues:

> "Old age should burn and rave at close of day;
> Rage, rage against the dying of the light".
> (Whitaker, 1984 : 31)

And I say, if old age should "rage" at death, how much more

should someone at my age (forty, as I write)? It's that increasing tension between suspecting that the dying process itself will be OK, and yet the feeling of terror at parting from those we love.

After all that, I am concerned again about under my left arm, though in all honesty, I can't find anything suspicious there. It could be just wear and tear, because all of me has got so out of condition with what has happened (I've been lifting heavy pots around for tea tonight and last weekend I drove the furthest I've driven yet, so my muscles are working more than they have been for a while), but there's just this nagging feeling; and in the scar of my neck, it feels tender and Jeremy and I have both wondered if we've felt a very tiny 'pea' there. But it's been tender most of the time, it could equally be scar tissue, or the final stages of my original lump disappearing – or growing again?

This is why I have to start to live in a different way. All this scares me as long as I am afraid of dying. The reality is that even if I eventually have a shortened life span because of my cancer, I am not going to die tomorrow or even next week, month or year. If the cancer should come again soon, there are other options apart from the Arimidex. One being chemotherapy, and that worked last time. I had four and a half years of remission last time. How might cancer treatments have advanced in another four and a half years? I want that much time to get Katie to the stage that Jamie is now, so I know she would be able to cope if I had to leave.

This hurts such a lot to look at. It makes me grief stricken and I am reminded of Elizabeth Barrett Browning's poem "Grief", in which she writes:

> "I tell you, hopeless grief is passionless;
> That only men incredulous of despair,

Half-taught in anguish, through the midnight air
Beat upward to God's throne in loud access
Of shrieking and reproach. Full desertness
In souls as countries, lieth silent bare
Under the blanching, vertical eye-glare
Of the absolute Heavens."
(Norris, 1991 : 73)

Was that me last time I had active cancer? Incredulous, therefore able to shriek and protest to God, that this could not possibly be happening to me. This time, I have almost felt myself – till now – to be hanging in suspension, incapable of relationship with God, just like the poem's statue in the immobility/stupor of grief. Somehow, I feel led to look at all this. It's as though I have to surrender a lot this time, to be able to live what's left well. Why have I always put myself under pressure? If I start allowing life to be easier for myself, my body will be able to take care of its own healing, rather than struggling against the pressure I put on it that leads to the exhaustion that decimates me. Why am I so hard on myself? I am the person who has the highest expectations of myself.

Into this equation, comes the question about whether to even think about taking up my Masters Degree again. Might that also be pressure on me that is actually unnecessary?

Kathy Keay was studying for a doctorate in women's spirituality at Bristol, when her first book was published in 1994. By the time her next book was published in 1996, her friend had to finish editing it, because she had died of breast cancer at the age of forty. I don't think it is possible for women to do everything in life. That is a fallacy. The working women, who get high in public office, or any other job, have nannies looking after their children. I have chosen both to work and to have time to give to the children. I can't study as well. I have no regrets about the times I've disengaged from study for the sake of the children. I think maybe this is another time to disengage. What will be achieved by a Masters Degree from Oxford University? I am not going to be a reliable employment risk for any new employer for a long time to come, if ever. I think I have to start getting my priorities right and remove the pressures from myself.

Maybe God could help me more if I lifted pressures and accepted help (even) more. It is the lesson I am learning very much this time – to accept help. And in that context it was very reassuring at the weekend to have the experience of feeling Jennifer (our daughter, still born at 34 weeks) was behind Katie. I have always thought of her as my Guardian Angel. She obviously looks out for Katie as well and, therefore by inference, Jamie too and Jeremy. That is very reassuring and takes pressure off me, if ever I can't be here for them all. Also reassuring is the feeling that God still believes in me, despite all my doubts and fears.

"METHODIST RECORDER" ARTICLE, 8 NOVEMBER 2001

★

We are a manse family (living in a church house) with two rapidly growing children. Katie (10) is an avid fan of The Simpsons, so over the years, I have come to know a thing or two about Homer, Marge and the rest of the family. As I approached the end of my tenth year in the ministry of the Methodist Church, it was Homer's catch phrase, "Mmmm doughnuts!" that started buzzing round my head. Except that in my case, the words became, "Mmmm sabbatical!"

I was really looking forward to my sabbatical, and to be honest, I thought I deserved it. After my first appointment in rural Lincolnshire (six churches in six different communities), we had moved to the Midlands, with a sense of anticipation, as I took on the responsibilities of Superintendent Minister of a group of eight churches and their staff, as well as the pastoral care of three of those churches. I've tried to work hard throughout that period; like anyone else I've made my mistakes, but like many other ministers, I have been held and affirmed in the job I do by the love and care of the Methodist people, whom it has been my privilege to serve. Still, there have been times when the work has been hard and demanding, so the gift of a sabbatical on my horizon was a wonderful thought. Time to continue research for my dissertation, to rest a bit, to travel.

I was careful to arrange cover for all my work, booked flights for my son and myself to Texas for 17th April 2001, and looked forward with anticipation to receiving my just desserts... Then I went for my annual check-up with the surgeon who first diagnosed that I had simultaneous breast cancers in December 1996 (just after we arrived in the Midlands). After chemotherapy and a bilateral mastectomy, I had recovered my health and strength and was well on track for the magical five years clear of cancer from date of diagnosis. Now it was Maundy Thursday 2001. I told my consultant that I had just found a pea-sized lump in the nape of my neck (in the days before my appointment); and he told me that if I came into hospital on Easter Tuesday, he would operate and take a biopsy on the Wednesday. I said that I was supposed to be flying out to Texas that day. He said, "I wouldn't if I were you."

The next bit we are intensely proud about, for our son Jamie (fifteen) decided that he would take the ten hour flight to Dallas/Fort Worth by himself to stay with our friends there, as he knew there was a risk I would lose all the monies that had gone into our planning if he didn't. I kept hoping I would be able to go and join him; but my biopsy results showed a return of the breast cancer I'd had previously, and so began the round of scans that you are given to discover the full extent of your cancer. To cut a long story short, an ultrasound scan revealed a cyst on my right ovary, which had to be checked out, before I could receive my cancer treatment. So, one Monday I met a gynaecologist who specializes in cancer and he told me that if I went into hospital the next day, he would operate on the Wednesday. We decided on a complete hysterectomy (plus my ovaries), and decided against any neat little bikini cut, because a larger, more old-fashioned incision would enable him to have a good look round my stomach cavity whilst he was at it.

The good news was that my cyst (actually discovered to be on my womb) was benign, my ovaries were normal and there was no other cancer to be seen elsewhere in my stomach. As far as it is possible to tell, my only tumour was the one in my neck. So, as a result, I am able to take a hormone tablet that wasn't available when I was ill last time (and for which you have to be post-menopausal) to block the "keyholes" in my tumour, so that oestrogen still being produced by my adrenal glands can't fit in there and help it to grow – my cancer is of the hormone-receptive type. The even better news is that (since my hysterectomy and starting my medication), my tumour has gone and I am again in remission from my cancer.

Meanwhile, I have been off work for the last five months, and am now trying to adjust to life again after recurrence of cancer and a major operation, that hurled me (at forty) straight into the menopause. There are humorous sides to my situation. For instance, I am not sure how I will ever preach again to the particular member of my congregation who quite unexpectedly (on a normal morning working as a theatre nurse) found herself assisting in my operation – what do you say to someone who has seen even more of you than you have ever seen yourself?! And as winter approaches, and the family huddle into their winter woollies, what will we all do when Mum has to strip off virtually to her underwear and open every door and window in sight to relieve hot flushes? It may be true, as my son pointed out to me, "Real women don't have hot flushes – they have power surges". But what if I have a "power surge" in the pulpit? The mind boggles!

I have to say that it has been a bit of a struggle – for my family and me – to cope with cancer a second time in our lives. I have kind of viewed God from a distance for a while – not because I have ever had cause to doubt God's Presence in life, but because I have found myself asking very hard questions about the nature of that God. They're not new questions, lots of people have asked them before me (even as far back as the writer of the book of "Job" in the Old Testament of the Bible), but they're still hard to struggle with, even though I began to tackle them somewhat when Jennifer was stillborn in 1987. Yet in all my grief and fury about the things that have happened to me since Easter, I know for sure that I have been upheld by the grace of God, though not necessarily as a result of my own faith, for at times that flame has flickered very low. Instead, I have been upheld by the love and faith of my family, friends and colleagues, and most of all by the people in the churches of the Black Country, many of whom say to me, "I pray for you every night" – and I know that they do. Their kindness and compassion has been of immeasurable comfort to me.

This has been underlined for me since I lit a ring of candles in my private devotions earlier this week, and realised that although the centre candle was not alight, it was illumined by the light from the candles round about it. I am grateful to God for surrounding me with the light of the faith of so many people during a very hard time in my life; and I pray that as I continue to get well, I may help God's Spirit to build the kind of community where each person may be held and loved in their time of need, until they are able to reach out a hand of faith and friendship to the people who struggle with life's hard questions on either side.

THINKING ON THE WRITING OF
KATHY KEAY

★

In "After Breast Cancer Diagnosis April 1993", Kathy Keay wrote:

> "Prayer is a silence and a shouting
> a burst of praise
> a thanksgiving
> welling up and out of us
> in spite of everything."
> (1996: 127)

In "God Is With Us", she went on to say that:

> "God is with us, through loneliness, bereavement, broken relationships and unemployment, as well as at times of great joy and achievement. Nothing can surprise or shock God. He knows and deeply loves each of us. Once we understand this we can live life to the full, even against impossible odds."
> (1996: 129)

Whilst I acknowledge the presence of God enabling us to live life to the full, I am wondering whether God is one that will express relationship with the individual, and whether the relationship is to be described as one of LOVE? However, I am fully with Kathy

Keay in her recognition of the fact that a gift, which comes alongside illness, is time to slow down and see life. As she writes in "The Grass Is Greenest":

> "In reality, the grass is greenest where we water it most, and there is so much to live for − if we have the eyes to see − the smile of a small child, a blaze of colour from a bunch of flowers, or the spontaneous comment which lifts our spirits and makes us laugh. All are life's gifts and signs of God's unshakeable commitment to us."
> (1996: 150)

JOURNAL
27 NOVEMBER 2001

★

Asked if I would write a letter for the church's Christmas magazine, I found myself at rather a loss about what to write, as I feel that I am in a kind of "in-between place" at the moment: *"In-between" Easter and the rapid approach of Christmas...* Having been "signed off" right after Easter (seven months ago), and hoping to do A FEW things to get back into work before Christmas, I feel very much better physically and mentally at the moment – thanks to the EXCELLENT care I have received from my own G.P. and Newcross Hospital and the time a very able counsellor has given me through the anonymity of the Churches' Ministerial Counselling Service. And thanks also to all the love, support and friendship received from so many people over such a long period of time.

"In-between" who I was and who I one day will be... People say to me, "you mustn't overdo it, when you come back to work". I don't think they understand, that I WON'T BE ABLE to overdo it! I am not the same person as I was, before I experienced the recurrence of cancer in my life – either mentally or physically. I am going to continue to discover who I am, but folks may have to get used to me saying, "no, I can't do that," and I certainly don't intend to be taking back responsibilities that other folk have carried out so ably in my absence. As far as I can see, folk have all made an excellent job of being the church in the places where

they live without me. I'm sure that there's still work for me to do, but certainly in the beginning, preaching, worship preparation and some pastoral work will be about all I can manage, with plenty of rest "in-between" (there are those strange words again!).

"In-between" life and death (as indeed we all are)... I hope to live a long and useful life, if I am able so to do, but I have come to a new place, where I recognise that people don't just either "recover from" or "die of" cancer these days. There are hundreds, if not thousands of people like me, who will probably be cancer patients for the rest of their lives – who "live with" controlled disease. And I can tell you this much – there becomes nothing so sweet as the PRESENT MOMENT in these circumstances (which is, after all, all that any of us are actually guaranteed), and the colour of the light at a particular moment, or the time spent with your pet, your friend or a family member suddenly becomes more precious than you might be able to imagine. What was it that Jesus said to his friends, "in-between" his own birth and death, according to the gospel writer, St. Luke?

> "Can any of you by worrying add a single hour to your span of life? If then you are not able to do so small a thing as that, why do you worry about the rest? ....Do not keep striving for what you are to eat and what you are to drink, and do not keep worrying...your Father knows that you need them. Instead, strive for his kingdom, and these things will be given to you as well." [Luke 12:25-31, NRSV]

LETTER TO A FRIEND
3 DECEMBER 2001

★

The hard part (for all of us) comes in recognizing that death is also part of the (created) cycle, and that prayers can be just as much answered if life ends, when we would rather it didn't. However, I have learnt this year that breast cancer can be lived with these days as a 'controlled' disease. This has brought a big and helpful change to my mindset. Although I am not intending to 'shuffle off this mortal coil' anytime in the near future, I know that when I do (whenever that may be), the act of dying must also be part of the created order that is (in itself) part of God.

In this respect, I find the writing of W.H. Vanstone useful at the moment. My colleague found his book, "Love's Endeavour, Love's Expense", helpful and he bought it for me at the beginning of this second-time around illness. As I've said before, I have always have believed that there is a right time to read a book! I am overlooking the exclusive language (this once!) as the book was first published in 1977 and (according to the blurb), Vanstone "is one of a brilliant post-war generation of Anglican theologians" who "unlike many of his contemporaries... turned aside from the writing of books and the taking up of academic appointments to commit himself unreservedly to the life of a parish priest in a housing estate in the north of England...." More power to his elbow!!

Vanstone takes the image of an artist, who is always seeking to stretch his powers to (and even beyond) their limit, so that by engaging them to the utmost, he enlarges his own artistic capacity. Vanstone goes on to suggest that, at the moment when the artist exceeds his known powers, his new work (be it painting or poem) balances precariously between "triumph and tragedy" (p.47). There is, in fact, a moment when the whole work is out of balance and if the artist was to be interrupted at that point, his creation would undoubtedly be marred by an "excess of boldness" (p.48).

Instead, Vanstone suggests, that it can be at he very moment when the painting or poem looks as though it will fail, that the artist may triumph by developing his excess in such a way that his work now has an extra dimension. So that, in actual fact, the risk-taking leads to a work of genius, which comes from the willingness of the artist to risk losing control of his creation:

> "We see, at the moment of lost control, the most intense endeavour of the artist: and his greatness lies in his ability to discover ever-new reserves of power to meet each challenge of precarious adventure – each challenge of powers exceeded and control lost. As we follow, in actuality or retrospect, the fashioning of a work of art, we are always conscious of it as poised upon the brink of failure... Each decisive step is a precarious step, to be redeemed from tragedy only by the next and equally precarious step, of correction or new discovery, which must be improvised to succeed it." (1998 : 48)

I would argue for such a moment of lost control in creation, when its beauty could have been marred by the disfigurement of diseases like cancer, for instance. Instead, the brushstroke which redeems that apparent "excess" (to use Vanstone's terminology) and shows that God the Creator continues the work of creation and was never (in fact) interrupted from it, is that which extends divine creativity to men and women, so that they are able to discover ways to combat and even (sometimes) cure dreadful diseases.

EMAIL TO IAN, 18 DECEMBER 2001

★

Dear Ian – Thank you for all your good wishes. I am feeling particularly down this evening, so it was nice to find your email. Waiting to have an aspiration (needle in neck to collect cells), as I think that the lump is regrowing in my neck (have I told you this?). If it is cancer again, chemo after Christmas. I am pissed off. I think I have told you this. It seems such a long time this time. Grief is bad at times. It's good that I seem well apart from the lump – i.e. no cancer symptoms elsewhere; good that its five years since I last had chemo... bad that it could be because cancer has become unstable that it's come back – i.e. has adapted and learned to grow despite my hysterectomy and the Arimidex both helping to block oestrogen. If it weren't in me, I'd probably think that it was a clever little bastard. I am trying to do a few things to keep my mind busy, but have to allow lots of rest time. Can't begin to enunciate the exhaustion that comes with this bloody thing in emotional terms. Having said that, you probably have a fair idea, if you compare it to your depression.

Hope you are feeling a little better. Sam must be good for you. Sophie seems good for me. She has obviously come to stay (have I told you about her?). A much traumatised dog – obviously knocked about by a man, as she dislikes men very much, but we have finally got all her weeing and pooing out of doors, though it does mean me and/or Jeremy getting up in the night. She seems to think that I am the cat's whiskers! Cats' whiskers are out of joint, but they have shown no sign of leaving or being so upset that dog has to go. I think she was "sent" – to exercise me and take my mind off me.

Re the poem you sent ("Christmas" by John Betjeman) – it's lovely, but do you still believe that God tipped Godself completely into a person? I don't think that it's possible, though I accept that Jesus walked very close to God. Would I be cast out as a heretic if this was publicised?! Here is one of my favourite seasonal poems in return, by Thomas Hardy, which comes with love and licks from Sophie – though she probably sends some growls to Sam, because she doesn't seem to like dogs any more than she likes men. Think she must have been harassed in her first season, which vet thinks she has had. Hopefully no puppies on the way!! Only time will tell.

Love from Lesley XXX

"Christmas Eve, and twelve of the clock.
'Now they are all on their knees,'
An elder said as we sat in a flock
By the embers in fireside ease.

We pictured the meek mild creatures where
They dwelt in their strawy pen,
Nor did it occur to one of us there
To doubt they were kneeling then.

So fair a fancy few would weave
In these years! Yet, I feel,
If someone said on Christmas Eve.
'Come; see the oxen kneel.

In the lonely barton by yonder coomb
Our childhood used to know,'
I should go with him in the gloom,
Hoping it might be so."
(Philip, 1990 : 111)

LETTER TO JOSE 8 JANUARY 2002

★

Dear Jose – How are you? We have been thinking of you such a lot since we received your last letter on Christmas Eve. How are you now? Did you decide to let your lawyer try for clemency or look for any problems in the law regarding your case? I too have been waiting, waiting... I had an aspiration on 27 December. I have managed to find out the results of that today. It is the cancer growing again in my neck, but that is not a surprise for me, because I knew in myself that that was the case. So I see my oncologist (cancer doctor) again on Friday (11 January), and expect to start a course of chemotherapy next week. I must be hopeful and positive. As it is five years since I last had any chemotherapy, and as it was the chemotherapy that got rid of the cancer last time for me, it will hopefully work for me again. It works by damaging the DNA in the cancer cells, so that when they go to reproduce, they self-destruct instead. It is a shame that the hormone therapy hasn't given me a longer remission; but it gave me time to recover from my big operation, so I should be able to cope with chemotherapy better now than if I had it straight after a big operation. I have discovered that the reason that the hormone treatment is now less effective is probably because the cancer cells have found a way to grow, despite the fact that they have been "starved" of the oestrogen that feeds my kind of cancer.

In myself, I am feeling fairly fit again – having a dog keeps me fit, because she has to be walked a couple of times a day! She is some kind of collie/whippet cross; and if I tell you that collies are bred as working dogs, and round up the sheep for the farmers on hill farms, and whippets are bred to race, you will realise that she can run VERY fast! She has obviously been mistreated and had to sit still for long periods of time, so the more she gets used to running, the more she will need to run, I expect. But I don't mind, me walking and her running is very good for both of us! And it makes me laugh when I try to run with her, and she runs VERY slowly to keep me company. I say to her, "Sophie, you don't have to make it so obvious that you are politely trying to keep an old lady company!!"

Anyway, it means that physically I am feeling fairly fit. It has been the mental strain of waiting for things to happen...tests, results and so on that is wearing me out. But then I don't have to tell you about any of that. I just try and look at your patience in coping with a much worse situation of torture, and see what I can learn from you – so you see, we are good for each other, our friendship is not just a one-way benefit!! Therefore, I really don't want to lose your friendship, so I feel very angry and upset, when I think that that might be going to happen sometime in the near future.

I rang up Rachel at Lifelines. She said she had six execution dates (when I rang her) between now and Easter. She said that if George W. Bush had still been Governor, she would have expected to have twelve by Easter, but that it was still taking time to see how things are going to work out under the new Governor, even though he is pro-death penalty. What a system! It is hard for many of us to understand how the man who is now seen as the most powerful in the world, can have signed so many death warrants in his time as Governor of Texas.

I do want to try and come and see you, but things are a bit different now, as I know you would be the first to tell me. I have to find out from my cancer doctor what kind of treatment I have to have, and talk to him about coming to see you. I asked the nurse and she said that she didn't think there would be a problem with me wanting to go to the States, as your medics are well up on cancer treatment there. She said she would probably tell me not to go to some other countries in the world, but I know you will understand that I have to think of myself first. If I don't do that at this stage in my life, I won't be able to be of help to any of my family or friends in the long run.

So what this means is, that I may not be able to come and be with you, if you get a date set, as I hoped previously to do. This is because I think that if I can come, it will have to be in the next six weeks or so. If I have the same type of chemo as before (one dose every three weeks, for six doses), I know that in the days after a dose, I don't feel brilliant, and then I have two weeks where I feel fairly well before the next dose. But as the effect is cumulative, by the end, I will feel not so good for a while, until my body recovers. So, I would need to come sometime during the first two treatments, as after that the journey would be too long and tiring for me. I will talk to the doctor on Friday and see what he says. Meanwhile, if you have any more information, let me know. Am I still on your visiting list any way? What I am saying is maybe I can just come and visit you, like I planned to do last Easter before all this happened to both of us.

I have also asked a friend if he would be able to come with me to Texas, as I wouldn't come on my own at the moment (I would if I was 100% fit). He says he will let me know, but it may be that he and his wife would both come; which means that I would have company on the long flight (you know I don't like flying!)

and he could do the driving once we are out there. So I could have a little bit of that holiday that I missed last year, and also see our friends in Dallas once again, which I would love to do. We must both keep thinking and praying about the situation. I feel sure that if it is to be possible for me to see you again, it will all work out; whereas, we both know that God will give us the patience and endurance we need, if that is not to be so.

I think that we must have both learnt a lot in the patience and endurance stakes in these last five years! I say to people I am both more patient and less patient than I used to be! More patient, because I can wait and take time to make decisions these days, where a younger me would have had to get things worked out immediately. More patient, just because I know that time keeps moving and things always get worked through in the end, whether I rush around and try to sort them or not. Less patient, because I get really bugged these days by people who get all agitated about things that really don't matter in the long run! And less patient, because it becomes more and more obvious to me that lots of people have lives they really have to struggle with (not just me and you!), while some people complain about nothing at all, in my estimation! Somehow, God seems to give us the strength to get on with it, though I have lots of questions I wish that God would answer for me! You have more patience and faith than me in that respect!

Jeremy is well and getting on well with his job, which is great. He has just had lunch and gone out to work, as he is on the 2-10pm shift this week. Katie doesn't like it, because she only sees him at breakfast time every day. She prefers the weeks that he is on the 6am-2pm shift. His work is obviously the reason that he would not be able to come out with me to Texas this time. Katie is well. Did I tell you that she has been offered a place at St.

Peter's, which is the school that Jamie goes to? So we are obviously very pleased about that. She starts there in September, as she is now eleven. It is hard to believe that soon both my children will be in Senior School!

Jamie is in the middle of mock examinations at school at the moment. They provide a practice run for the real exams, which sixteen year olds have to take in the summer term in this country. Jamie will be sixteen on March 25. How do I manage to believe that?! How can my son have grown so much? When I was at the Doctor's this morning, I was looking at a baby that was being bottle fed by its mother and thinking, "Was Jamie once that size?!" It seems unbelievable now! But he was and I am so grateful that I was able to have both my children (and feed them both myself until they were about ten months old), before all this happened to me and I lost all the parts that make having a baby and feeding a baby possible. I say to Jeremy that he should part-exchange me for a new model of wife!! But who would want this battered old person second-hand?! At least my family knows all about my amazing selection of scars and don't seem to be too much bothered about them.

The other thing I can't believe is the number of animals we have in our house these days. Actually it is very good for me. When I start feeling low, I have to see to cats, dog, guinea pigs or rabbit, and that takes my mind off me! Somebody the other day told me of her aunt, who used to say sometimes, "I've got PLOM's disease today. I'll be better tomorrow." That means "POOR LITTLE OLD ME!" I know that feeling. It is very destructive. When I know I am beginning to feel that way, that is when I look to friends or family or a quiet time for rescue! Well, my friend, I must sign off now. I want to have a bit of a lie down before I go and get Katie from school. I will post this on my way out.

EMAIL TO STELLA, MY COUNSELLOR, 25 FEBRUARY 2002

★

Dear Stella – Today S (Jamie's contemporary at S. Peter's) phoned to tell me that his Dad died on Saturday. Do you remember that I was feeling upset about T's cancer last week (I had visited him on the Tuesday)? I know that he knew his cancer was terminal, but I don't think that he expected to die quite so soon, as we were hoping to see each other when we went for treatment on Wednesday this week. I feel very sad about T's death. I liked him. He didn't deserve what he had dished out to him. I also feel troubled that a lad my son's age is obviously helping his Mum tell people that T has died. S doesn't deserve that either. But then that guy didn't deserve to have his throat cut on video in Afghanistan and his head chopped off after. Neither did all the Jewish victims of Eichman deserve what they received, nor did the guy Jeremy told me about deserve to be pushed onto a railway track and not be allowed to get off when a train was approaching by thugs. Such malevolent evil is hard to comprehend.

Today my friend Kath (the older lady that I met in hospital) also phoned me to say that she was feeling low, because she had been fitted in for an appointment with her oncologist today. She thinks her cancer is coming back in her tummy – and who am I to disagree? I know that we tend to know before our doctors what is going on in our bodies. I've just rung to see how she got on, but she's engaged on the phone. Another friend, Sue, rang to see if I could give her a lift to hospital for her bloods tomorrow. She had bloods taken last week and was borderline, so may not be able to have her treatment Wednesday. Apparently, when she saw Dr C last week, she had to have a chest X-ray and ultrasound scan to test her lungs and liver. Dr C is concerned that she is losing weight.

What should I do? Refuse to enter into relationship with anyone any more? The only way to cut out the pain of relationship, it seems to me, is not to enter into it. But then life would be infinitely less rich and tolerable. I wish T had been able to see his son again – he was longing for the 4th March, when that particular son would be home after working abroad. His other son also lives abroad and his daughter on the south coast. S was the only one still home with his parents.

Kath just rang. Her cancer has come back, and she has to have more aggressive chemo. She will lose her hair. Then I realise that I've already lost my hair...and (since I saw you) have had to go to hospital and am on triple antibiotics, because my blood count was low. So I have anti-bacterial, anti-viral and anti-fungal tablets to take. So I may not be able to have my chemo this week – depend on tomorrow's bloods.

I do feel better (though tired) after our mini break of a weekend away seeing Jeremy's folks and staying in a nice Travel lodge. But life is complicated, because I think I need a filling sorting out – suspect that's why I keep getting infections – they originate in my mouth. And I can't have any invasive dental work without my oncologist's say so. Still, we battle on. Good bits and bad bits to most days. At least I feel quite strongly prompted when I need to do things, which helps. I was prompted to phone and visit T last week. Today is quiet, so presumably the Prompter is giving me an unexpected day off, or a day to cope with my grief about my friends?

I am privileged that the church lets me continue to "work" – in any other context the amount I do would have meant I'd have been booted out long ago.

Still it certainly trains me well for living a day at a time and enjoying the good days when they arrive. Thanks for listening and for the crystallised ginger, which stops me feeling sick – yum!
Lesley X

ARTICLE FOR "THE METHODIST RECORDER", 28 FEBRUARY 2002

★

> "Our help is in the name of the eternal God, who is making the heavens and the earth."

Thus runs Jim Cotter's paraphrase of Psalm 124, verse 8 (1994 : 2). It is a phrasing to which I cling, because it speaks of the continuing presence of God in the world, despite a chaos, which (at times) threatens to subsume me. Chaos, which has come into my life through personal experience of life-threatening disease and indirect experience of the inhumanity, which seems sometimes to mark our human condition.

Having previously testified to my experience of breast cancer ("Recorder", 8 November 2001), I do not intend to go into much further detail, except to say that I recently began a course of chemotherapy to attempt (once again) to put into remission the cancer that has returned in my neck, after the brief respite provided last year by hormone therapy. Hopefully, chemotherapy will be as successful as it first was five years ago in attacking my 'despicable' disease (not the word I usually use to describe my cancer – but Methodist ministers are generally expected to be polite in public).

That was back in the days of my naïveté, when I ignorantly

thought that you either recovered from or died of cancer – not realising how many hundreds of people live active lives with a controlled disease. So I am currently receiving toxic injections, at least one of which works on the principle of so damaging the DNA in my cancer cells that they will be unable to reproduce when the time comes, and from their self-destruction will appear my remission. However, as I cope with my injections, I find that therein lies perplexity for me...

For I have a friend (of five years' standing) who lives several thousand miles away in the North American state of Texas, who, as I write, is also awaiting an injection of drugs, but the drugs for which he waits are intended to kill him. I started writing to Jose in the days of my recuperation from illness the first time round, because (after all) letter-writing is easy for me to do and can be fitted into the awkward-sized spaces of time that count as leisure for the average circuit minister. By the time I realised that it is not 'easy' to undertake relationship with a man on Death Row, I was far too committed to turn back and the rest, as they say, is history. Suffice here to say that Jose has become a member of our family and a dearly loved friend, who has enlarged my life experience no end and changed me irrevocably as a person and as a Christian.

I managed to visit Jose in the maximum-security prison near Huntsville, Texas, two years ago; and would have gone again last year in my sabbatical, if illness had not intervened. Now I am wondering if I will be able to see him again before he is killed though my consultant seems to think that we may be able to fit in such a visit with my chemotherapy schedule should the need arise. The thing is, after ten years on Death Row, Fifth Circuit (almost the final level of appeals procedure, apart from the Supreme Court) has denied Jose's appeal. He has not yet received an execution date, but unless his lawyer can find anything finally to help his case, such a date looks fairly inevitable. The minimum statutory notice for setting such a date is thirty days and, even after five years, I have never grown accustomed to the fact that, in Texas, dates to kill men and women seem to be set in as routine a way as those which we might set up to visit the doctor or dentist in our own country...

My perplexity is in no way lessened when I consider that the man who is now considered the most powerful in the world (George W. Bush, a member of the United Methodist Church, which holds a position anti-death penalty) has, in his time as Governor of Texas signed somewhere more than one hundred and fifty death warrants, which I suspect may be more than any state governor in the USA this century.

As the chaos of my own cancer and my friend's (increasingly imminent) execution whirl around me, I sometimes find it hard to discern God in the reality of my life experience. Some days I feel caught between two (opposing?) points if view. "The Prayer of Jabez", a little book by Bruce Wilkinson, in parts helpfully expounds an almost obscure verse from the First Book of Chronicles in the Bible, when Jabez implores God, "Oh, that you would bless me indeed..." I can see eye to eye with that, but, on the other hand, I am often more impressed with the little bookmark bearing the observation of one penguin to his friend, who is being eaten by a giant fish, "Relax, God's in control!"

As I have previously suggested, it is undoubtedly the nature of God with which I tussle these days; more perhaps than with doubt of God's presence – though I would never have come this far in this particular battle if God had not invested physical presence for me in the personalities of my family, friends, colleagues and local church members and friends. Many times,

50

they have pulled me back from the abyss that has threatened to engulf me.

Yet, through everything, I am impressed by my friend Jose's unwavering faith in God and the reality of the relationship that he has undoubtedly maintained with God over the five years that I have known him. Jose seems sure that, whilst almost everyone else has given up on him, God forgives and loves him and therefore, he is in no way afraid to die. I dare to hope that God has been able to communicate through me and those of my friends and family who now write to Jose some of the love that is often most easily expressed through physical personality, but not always, as Jose's closeness to the invisible Spirit of God testifies. I wonder whether such faith as he possesses even so close as he must now be to Death Watch can also be true for me? Despite my cancer? Or even because of it?

I find rest in some hopeful words of R.S. Thomas, that maverick Welsh clergyman, who, it seems to me, fought a fierce faith battle most of his life. He wrote:

> "I think that maybe
> I will be a little surer
> of being a little nearer.
> That's all. Eternity
> is in the understanding
> that that little is more than
> enough."
> (1990 : 63)

EMAIL TO PETER, 4 MARCH 2002

★

"It's my life, it's now or never, I ain't gonna live for ever, I just want to live while I'm alive...." Thus runs a line in a track from a 1995 Bon Jovi album (which incidentally, I intend to play at my 'do' in June). I need to write down some thoughts for clarity, but I write in the knowledge that you might have to excommunicate me, in your position within the Church hierarchy!

I am guessing that you were probably at T's funeral on Saturday. I was by the doorway in the lounge, and left relatively early on, because it was getting too crowded for me to sensibly stay, if I want my chemo tomorrow (I couldn't have my third dose last Wednesday, because my blood count wasn't high enough). I have been disturbed (as you may guess) by T's death. Also have felt the need to grieve for him, because I liked him. Incidentally, went to see him on the Tuesday before he died; so S (who's in Jamie's year at school) phoned me to tell me of his Dad's death ("no job for a fifteen year old, God", say I).

Now, as I say, I didn't see/hear much of the service, but I am troubled by what I did hear/see, in that I suspect we need an opportunity for endings, which I suspect a thanksgiving for life and love doesn't really provide. (Interesting that I'm having a thanksgiving in June – but I'm not dead ...yet.... nor will I be for some years to come, unless the effects of the treatment see me off, before the cancer itself does.) You see, sitting before the service with that big photo of T on the screen in front of me (as large as life, you might say), could have fooled me into thinking that T wasn't really dead – especially as (being in the church lounge) I couldn't see the coffin. And the minister, voicing T's comments, said that when he died, he didn't want a funeral, he wanted a party... well, um, forgive me, but I don't intend to celebrate dying... what comes next is too uncertain.

When Jennifer died (who, incidentally would have been fifteen last month) these verses from a poem by James Russell Lowell were too painful, but became very meaningful... You can find them in the anthology, "All in the end is harvest", edited by Agnes Whittaker:

> "Immortal? I feel it and know it,
> Who doubts it of such as she?
> But that is the pang's very secret, –
> Immortal away from me.
>
> Console if you will, I can bear it;
> 'Tis a well-meant alms of breath;
> But not all the preaching since Adam
> Has made Death other than Death.
>
> Communion in spirit! Forgive me,
> But I, who am earthly and weak,
> Would give all my incomes from dreamland
> For a touch of her hand on my cheek..."
> (1984 : 52)

I think what I'm trying to say, is yes, let's celebrate a life well-lived and let's be hopeful for the possibility of life after death, but we do need to acknowledge the loss of a person in the here and now, when they have died. S will go to school and come home to no Dad now. When everyone has left after the funeral, J will have no physical husband any more. I can't go and see T and chat and laugh and pray together any more, because he is dead now. And I grieve for that deadness, that loss to me...

More and more, I suspect our thoughts of heaven are to help us cope with the terrifying nature of this life. I don't know what paper you take, but Saturday's "Guardian" had, 'A vision of hell in Indian city gorging on violence' with a picture of a Muslim begging police for help as a Hindu mob surrounded his home.... On the news last night, there was a brief interview with a man who had only been able to save one small son, from the blaze onto which his entire family had been cast, before we were hurried on to Will, Pop Idol's success. I felt like rewinding the tape and saying to someone (who?), "Excuse me, did I just hear aright in that sound-bite that a man's sons were cast alive onto a fire?" I couldn't take it in. I said to Jeremy, "What would you have done if someone had thrown Jamie on a fire?" He said, "Kill them". I think I would too.

Then, last week, I read somewhere about two thrones in heaven; the thrones of mercy and judgement. Where are these thrones suspended? What space in the ethereal heavens accommodates them? In the light of all I've said above, I can see the need of people to believe in this kind of story – it deals with our fears about what happens after our own death, and it neatly tidies up for us all the horror of this world, because God will sort all the baddies out on the other side. But it is meaningless to me.

Incidentally, I just purchased from Methodist Publishing House a book by Barbara Baisley called "No Easy Answers: An Exploration of Suffering". It's about her experience of breast cancer over the last fourteen years, first diagnosed when she was in her early thirties. I am going to try and read it, but there are two obstacles to beginning. The first is that, she starts her introduction with the words, "I have cancer – but that is not what this book is about, or rather, cancer is not the point..." which provides me with a supreme hurdle to cross, because the book is all about experiences which have come out of cancer, so who is denying what here?

Secondly, in his forward, the Bishop of Birmingham writes, "If we allow (God) to, he will use such experiences of suffering so that ultimately we can say, as Barbara did, that in whatever guise it comes, suffering is a peculiar, horrible and yet precious gift, transforming us into the people God wants us to be." The words I would use to explain my thoughts re this sentence are not printable to someone in your position of authority.

So, the struggle with this bloody disease, or rather (for me at the moment) the effects of the horrible treatment continue. I try and do a little work. I am grateful to the church for allowing this little. I know that I could not hold down a job in any other sphere of employment at the moment. The people with whom I work, are of inestimable value in helping me through this time of my life. To which end, I will conclude with some words from another Bon Jovi track (also to be played at my 'do'):

> "Thank you for loving me, for being my eyes when I couldn't see, for parting my lips when I couldn't breath...thank you for loving me." (1995)

EMAIL TO STELLA, MY COUNSELLOR, MARCH 2002

*

Hi Stella – I had my chemo last Tuesday in the end, so am in collapse system week. Overall doing OK, though today I am absolutely exhausted, so will be going very steady. The exhaustion is not just physical – this has been a very difficult week. I am cross, because I have just lost a day's work as a result of various things. Basically, I am pretty voiceless. My voice disappeared last night, and along came a sore throat and chest tightness instead. I've cracked under stress. Although I suspected I had lost my voice through stress, because this has never happened to me before and because of my situation re chemo, I had to go and be checked out today. The hospital staff were marvellous, and nobody said other than I was doing the right thing, but it's made for three sessions in various hospitals this week, instead of two, and a day where I couldn't do my couple of carefully planned tasks, because of the need to rest.

At least the blood tests today showed that my bloods have already risen well after last week's chemo – they weren't low. A delightful doctor thoroughly checked my chest, and so on and could find no infection; so told me to use my judgment if I thought matters were deteriorating and get back to them for antibiotics if I needed them. I've had a lot in the last few weeks, so I was glad not to have them unnecessarily. And I can rest a stress-lost voice, as long as I know that's what it is. But when I get my first decent chemo experience out of three, which I've physically coped with well, I don't want to be emotionally flattened just for a change.

So we have a lot of work to do tomorrow. Will I be able to have a bit longer than an hour, if necessary? Would it help if I came a bit earlier? I'm sure I'll manage the drive, though you know I have to manage my time and energy whilst on treatment. At the moment I need to focus on getting well. Hopefully, I can help make things clearer tomorrow. Body allowing, I shall come, even if I do have to whisper. Any observer would think that Jeremy and I are part of the Klu Klux Klan at the moment, as all I do is whisper to him!

Yours,
Lesley

EMAIL TO ALISON, 16 MARCH 2002

Dear Alison – Yes please, we would very much like to see you next weekend. I should be fine, as my third chemo was 5 March (a week delayed) and therefore my next one is due 26 March. Physically, I have done brilliantly this time, though obviously still have to go steady; but am just ending a mega-bad week stress wise. Friends have been amazing, picking up the stressed-out mess of me. I cannot deal with this. In case no one noticed, I have cancer (had cancer) and am now bald through chemo. Actually, it would be easy to feel sorry for myself, but I won't allow it.

In the same week, my friend whose breast cancer, having spread to her bones ten years ago, has been controlled for that length of time, has discovered that it has gone to her liver and the specialist says she's got six to twelve months to live, eighteen months maximum (at the age of forty-four). My other friend (who I met in hospital) is struggling with recurrence of her bowel cancer and another friend went home to find men from the forces in her front room with her husband. Her navy son (twenty-nine next week) was killed in a diving accident. I cannot even begin to comprehend the horror. I would rather die myself (definitely) than ever be told that Jamie was dead. I would instantly fall to a million pieces and refuse to speak to God again. Sorry about this. I knew I was angry, but you don't deserve all the shit hurled at you! Never mind. I will survive. Hope your toe is soon better. Love, Lesley X

MONDAY 18 MARCH 2002

★

This morning when I woke up, I found that I was lying flattened on the bed, feeling (literally) like I had been run over by a steam-roller. Last night (after a lovely, but very long day) with our friends Jackie, Becky and their dog Sophie (yes, two 'Sophie' dogs!), I got to bed, realizing that I had overdone it with my voice and, as has happened each night on going to bed since I lost it, I nearly coughed my innards up. It was so painful in my throat and breathing tube, but I feel all right apart from that. Jackie had chemotherapy five years ago and is very supportive towards me. She came to get me from Grantham, when I needed a break after my biopsy last Easter, when I wasn't even capable of being put on a train here and collected the other end, let alone drive to her house (as I would usually do).

I think Sophie was sent to show me what unconditional love is like. She lies with her head on my lap, and gazes at me in adoration, whether I am wigged, capped, bald, slavering, coughing, whatever! I don't want people to adore me, but it is nice to be at least liked! I am not generally in the habit of not-liking people myself, though sometimes I feel frustrated or exas-perated by things they do. I try always to be careful in listening to what people say, because my experience of town-centre ministry (among the very vulnerable and needy, including many ex-offenders) is that, sadly, you can't always trust people. However, bearing in mind that you always need to employ safeguards in pastoral ministry, I nevertheless quite like even some of the rogues I meet, though I wouldn't trust them as far as I could throw them (which is no distance at all in my present condition!)

It is *very hard* to cope with the physical burden of myself at the moment. My bum hurts when I go to the toilet (piles and constipation combined) – I need cream for that. My mouth and throat get sore – I need mouthwash for that. My hands crack and my nail beds get damaged (I need rubber gloves, antiseptic cream, hand-cream for that). I am bald, which incidentally means I have no hair, because I have cancer. Actually I could die. I am reminded of John Diamond again:

> "... there are chapters of what you've read so far where I could accurately describe my state of mind only by adding the words 'and the thing is, I might die!' to the end of every sentence and having it printed in a 16-point Hysterical typeface..." (1999: 175)

Did manage two pieces of work today – meeting with local Vicar to catch up on our churches, and to plan future work together. Meeting with active retired man and new lay worker to see what particular work each of us were doing re my churches. That was enough for today. Now I am putting this journal to bed, and will have a quiet, non-talking evening; as I had another attack of the dreadful cough, when I was getting Katie's tea. It is quite frightening and gut wrenching. I am sure it is stress. It only happens when I've been using my voice too much, so I must rest it. I don't want to end up with an asthma attack. I am very aware that asthma can be stress-related...

EMAIL TO IAN, 19 MARCH 2002

★

Dear Ian – I have to say that I don't know whose life is the more unbelievable at the moment – yours or mine, but maybe we should just call it quits. I am afraid that you will not hear pastorally from others. My first article in "The Methodist Recorder" led to a small, but interesting selection of responses, presumably because I explained that I was still in the faith body due to the faith of others, and was hopeful that I was in remission from my cancer via hormone therapy. My second article has elicited no response, except one letter. But there I talked of being on the brink faith-wise, and having to have more treatment for recurring cancer, and linked my injections to the one Jose is awaiting (designed to kill him). I think that I was acknowledging too much pain, grief and doubt. The only response was from a retired minister, who has been very supportive recently, but then he is someone who knows about getting through grief and pain and muck. He knows life can be hard and so recognizes the pain of another person (though I reckon he deals with it all much more graciously than me). Many Church people don't seem to think that ours is the 'appropriate' reaction to the grief of life and say nothing, unless they don't see where we are coming from. Maybe that's why we have got on so well since regaining email contact – we know where each other is coming from. My main consolation is that the fewer and fewer people I find to be on the same path as me are greatly supportive and understanding.

I have just claimed the emergency appointment this afternoon at my Drs, having first consulted the staff at the hospital. Last week, I lost my voice through stress (which I have NEVER done before) and am suspecting I am developing an asthmatic kind of a cough to go with it. I won't bore you with all the details, just keep on, keeping on. Will be praying that the right path for your future will become evident to you. Sometimes it can't be revealed till you're off the path that is obscuring the view.

Love and Prayers,

Lesley XX

EMAIL TO STELLA, MY COUNSELLOR, 19 MARCH 2002

★

Dear Stella – Help! I think I may be sending up distress flares. Some people seem to be finding it hard to take on board the stuff that I have had to grapple with in this last year – the reality of my life/death as a cancer patient. I cannot take the blame for not being clearer about it myself, because I have been struggling enough with all that has happened to me. I can't sort it all out for everybody else as well. Maybe that is just what I have tried to do too often in my life at too high a cost. Sometimes, I get close to feeling very sorry for myself, in terms of "What have I done to deserve all this?" But then, what <u>have</u> I done to deserve all this? Just tried to act with integrity – and along come cancer and emotional trauma as a result. Gee whiz, God, so much for integrity in work and professional life! Don't tell me Jesus died as a result of trying to maintain his integrity! I don't know that I really want to accept that thought which has just popped into my head at this moment!

Lesley.

JOURNAL ENTRY, MARCH 2002

★

Time for some perspective?! I was originally diagnosed (very unusually) with simultaneous cancers (rather than one cancer that had spread to the other breast), which had both spread into my lymph system, so that there were tumours under both my arms. Therefore, at my initial diagnosis, I suppose I was already a woman with secondary breast cancer, though I did not realise that at the time, and would not have been able to cope with that knowledge if I had somehow managed to take it on board.

Then, when the tumour developed in my neck, it was a recurrence of the original breast cancer, but in a different site, again revealing that I had secondary breast cancer. This is not recognised by the medical profession as a curable disease (yet), but it is quite clearly identified as a controllable one (I don't know whether this is yet true for other forms of cancer). The nurse-counsellor at the Deansley Centre says I could view it in the same kind of way as something like diabetes or rheumatoid arthritis; both serious diseases, which can still kill people, but which (by and large) can be lived with under control for very long periods of time – maybe even a full lifetime, in the terms by which we judge a full life-time.

Dad's Mum, Mabel, died of breast cancer at the age of thirty, but she lived in the days when there was not a lot that could be done to help you, if surgery was unsuccessful in limiting the spread of the disease and remember that breast cancer (by its very nature) is systemic. Fortunately, I do not live in my grandmother's time. The treatment for breast cancer is literally improving daily, and I have benefited (though only briefly) from hormone-drug induced remission that helped me to recover from my hysterectomy. Arimidex was not (I think) available five years ago, when I was originally treated for this disease, so who knows what may be available in five years time?

Other good things to celebrate are the fact that my cancer has not spread to my liver, lungs, brain or bones. It will not kill me in my neck. So, once through this period of treatment, I can be quite hopeful and positive that I will once again regain health and live a fairly normal, active life. I am not going to die this year or any time in the immediate future. The difference between now and five years ago, is that I will always see myself as a cancer patient now, even if the cancer never comes back and I live to be a very old lady (which is always possible given the general longevity of our families if they survive the various diseases that have struck folk down in our histories). This fits into much the same frame of reference as that of an ex-alcoholic, who will generally refer to themselves as a "recovering" alcoholic, even if it is twenty or thirty years since they last touched a drop of liquor – because they know that they always have the potential to revert to being an alcoholic, as I will always have the potential to have a recurrence of my cancer.

This is not negative thinking. It is fact. I have proved within myself that our state of mind contributes (or not) to our well-being. I have no intention of dying from cancer (if I can help it), but I have had to learn to live on a day-to-day basis, which precludes forward planning. It also means that I have a greatly enhanced enjoyment of every day living, and want to celebrate in the here and now. My 'do' on the first of June is to say thank you for the gift of life now. For today. And it is to say to God, that my thanks are not conditional on there being a future in the here and now, though I recognise that it is also important for cancer patients to have realistic goals to look forward to, whilst learning to live in the reality of the present moment.

I also want to thank God for eighteen years of marriage. Given the nature of my disease, I don't want to leave celebrations like this till set times (like, for instance, twenty-five years). I hope to be able to celebrate such anniversaries, but I may not be able to. And I do thank God for the marriage I have with Jeremy. He has been a constant source of support and enrichment in my life. As I have discovered more about my cancer over the last five years, I have invariably discovered that he already knew (through his scientific reading) the facts that I have gained, but (if they had the potential to distress me) has not told me of them, until I was ready to discover them for myself. I am greatly touched by the way he has known for so long the reality of the facts surrounding secondary breast cancer, but has chosen to carry them himself, rather than burden me with something I was not yet ready to hear. My current oncologist was not in the department in 1996. I asked him whether he thought I had done well to reach the five-year mark, given my original diagnosis. He said, "yes". I asked what he would have rated my chances of doing so, if he had been present for the original diagnosis. He said "50/50", so already, I am an example of what positive thinking and the power of prayer, alongside advances in medical science can do to redeem a difficult situation. We continue to live in that hope.

One of the reasons I sought a counsellor in the last year, was that I needed to talk through the implications of my disease and treatment and what I felt about death and dying, in a way that I never did five years ago. And I needed to be able to do this apart from Jeremy. We talk about virtually everything together, but I didn't want to go through with him all my feelings about the harder parts of my situation – because he has his own hard feelings to deal with already. It is hard enough to live full-time with a person in my situation. Every member of the family needs some time apart from me, and it, which is one of the reasons that it has been so good Jeremy getting his job. I try not to load close family with the full extent of my feelings about cancer – I only talk at any depth about these to people like Stella. I have a great deal of professional experience working with people who have cancer. It is quite different coping with the disease on a professional level, and coping with it yourself or for a member of your family.

JOURNAL, THURSDAY, APRIL 25 2002

★

"O give thanks to the Lord, for he is good; his
steadfast love endures for ever!
Out of my distress I called on the Lord; the Lord
answered and set me in a broad place.
With the Lord on my side I do not fear. What can
mortals do to me?
I was pushed hard, so that I was falling, but the
Lord helped me.
The Lord is my strength and my might; he has
become my salvation.
I shall not die, but I shall live, and recount the
deeds of the Lord.
The Lord has punished me severely, but he did not
give me over to death.
I thank you that you have answered me and have
become my salvation.
You are my God, and I will give thanks to you; you
are my God, I will extol you."
(Psalm 118, New Revised Standard Version Bible)

I live with controlled disease; and I can't go back on that, or get
away from that. Indeed, had I but realized it, I have lived with
controlled disease for five and a half years. And then I must have
had the disease for at least a period of time before I knew of its
existence. A lot has happened in that time. It's not just a case of

wishing something were not true, but rather acknowledging the inescapability of it having been true for so long; and there being no way so much life can be wound back and rerun (even if you wished it to be – and probably you don't). The intensity of living life knowing you live with controlled disease is sometimes very great. Wouldn't it have been better to live these last years in a kind of 'normal' way, with just the usual expectations of life? That was never an option.

In her novel, "The Pilot's Wife", Anita Shreve talks of "envelopes" of time – when time just seems to open or shut, become longer or shorter or unravel. When you sit in a length of space which is immeasurable, while the rest of the world clatters past in some kind of frenetic way, not realizing that the frenzy is surface; and that time loops and spools beneath that surface. At the moment, the last five years feel compressed, folded together like mountains under pressure; so that it seems no time at all since I was first diagnosed with simultaneous cancers; and the conversation with my oncologist yesterday holds similar terrors, disbelief and incredulity as first knowing I had breast cancer. Yet he didn't tell me anything I didn't know. He only answered the question that I wanted to ask him:

> "Is it, at least a possibility, that the cancer will not return?"
> "Yes, it is a possibility."
> "But it is perhaps not very likely?"
> "No, it is not very likely."

I am in what is termed (his words) "complete" remission, because the cancer is no longer palpable; and I do respond well to treatment, so I could even have "a very long" remission (I don't want to ask what he would consider to be a "long remission").

Yes, I have done well to get this far. Dr. C talked in terms of cancer patients being "self-selecting" – those who survive the disease, when quite a few others in their position would by now have died of it. The reality is that (given my initial diagnosis), I have survived a length of time, in which other women would have lost their fight with the disease. Why have I survived so long? Has God become my salvation, as the Psalmist says? If so, why only <u>my</u> salvation and not that of another person, who has fought an equally long and hard battle with disease? It is perplexing, because life feels so arbitrary, yet there is an emotional level at which the Psalm feels true for me.

"I shall not die but live," feels as though it is being spoken to me, rather than clutched at by me, as it would have been five years ago. Spoken to me, when actually I am in the stage of not believing this will be my reality, but rather suspecting that in some period of time – perhaps not very far away, I will die when this disease recurs in some way. And when the Psalm is read in its entirety, it speaks clearly of an earlier age in the spiritual/psychological development of a people when a very external god figure was invoked to save the people from the wars and perplexities that surrounded them; and if you were on the winning side, you were the goodies blessed by god, and if not, tough.

Yet, still the Psalm seems to be speaking to me of an Otherness that has continued alongside the growth in maturity of the people. The perceptions of the Other may have changed, the ways of describing/perceiving the Other likewise, but the Other remains. And the Other seems to be holding me (as always has been the case) safe. Why? The Other being Life-force, which is at times (like the present) so tangible that I can almost feel it holding me, surrounding me, pressing in on me from every side. Filling me, regrowing me. The wallflowers and the broom, the apple-blossom and the garden generally have held me this week. To look at a flower is to find strength, because it speaks of immanence and presence. I reckon that this is what will hold me/us when I/we die if we allow it.

There must be a way of dying built into the fabric of life, because death is so inescapable, even if I live this life for a great many years to come. Even if the cancer never returns, I still must die. That is the great unchangeable fact that probably I/we wish more than anything else was not the case. And part of the present grief is wishing that (for a respite period at least), I could re-enter the days of childhood/youth when there was not this recognition of dying, but open-ended planning for a future.

Kubler Ross has very diagrammatic notions of the path of grief, through periods like shock, denial, anger and so on. Whilst I see that there are recognizable shared experiences of grief, which follow such patterns, I think grief is much more as John (the hospital chaplain in Lincoln) once described it – chaotic. So that you loop in and out of these various feelings – sometimes you have gone a long way along the road and suddenly, you loop back or sideways or whatever into a pool of feelings, from which you thought you had moved on.

I expect I feel the grief again at the moment, because of the debilitating nature of the treatment I am undergoing; and the way my body is struggling to keep up (teeth breaking, veins protesting, fat/muscles/skin developing peculiar shapes and swellings, growing fat from steroids). Who am I in this situation? I consciously reconstruct myself on bad days, which means nail polish, earrings, lipstick, hats, clothes, that say, "I am still here". I do not necessarily know who I am, or where I am located in this body; but somewhere inside this unfamiliar shape, I still exist.

I sometimes wish I could get out, or change the way things are, but I'm stuck here. And yet, despite everything, my hair is fuzzing and starting to grow again – the urge towards life seems irrepressible, despite everything.

The urge seen in the likes of the wallflowers to continue just to be, to continue growing, living, dying, growing again. Inescapable life. And what fascinates me this time, is the way that (almost despite myself) I find the positive thoughts creeping up inside me, even when I feel most concerned about the future, thoughts like:

"you've already way outlived predictions",

"the cancer has never yet appeared anywhere that can kill you – despite the amount of time actually lived with secondary breast cancer – it has not yet appeared in major organs or bones",

"it is possible that radiotherapy will either provide a long lasting remission or contain the cancer within the area of my upper arm and neck",

"you are still here after developing early cancer – possibly at that genetic 80% risk".

All of these things suggest to keep trusting and going forward, instead of being bogged down in grief, but I believe the grief has to be felt to be contained, measured, moved past, incorporated – all these and more, yet none of them are true...

Intermission
May 2002 – September 2003

"I trace the rainbow through the rain,
And feel the promise is not vain,
That morn shall tearless be."

[George Matheson]

"REACHING FOR THE RAINBOW"

★

My second course of chemotherapy in six years came to an end
sometime in June 2002. It was followed by fifteen days of radiotherapy to my neck and shoulder area. Then followed a respite
from active cancer and its treatment for just over a year, a period
during which I recovered health and strength, as (to date) it had
mainly been the treatment for cancer, which had made me ill,
rather than the cancer itself.

I marked the end of my second phase of living with this disease
with a service in church, which was planned as a kind of Rite of
Passage, marking the end of a particular stage of my life, whilst
hopefully clearing the stage for new beginnings. It was called
"Reaching For The Rainbow" and I envisioned it as a liturgical
drama in four parts. We held it on Saturday 1 June 2002 at
2.30pm. I chose, as the theme of the service, Jim Cotter's trans-
lation of a verse from the Book of Psalms in the Bible:

> "Our help is in the name of the eternal God who is
> making the heavens and the earth."
> (Cotter, 1994 : 2)

OVERTURE

★

The service opened with the track "Heal Me" from the album by Ronan Keating (2000), played as a kind of Overture to the liturgical drama:

> "When things don't turn out right
> And it feels like you've lost the fight
> When things don't work out quite the way
> Friend you can look my way...
> Chorus – Why won't you... heal me
>   Love won't you... steal me
>   Into the night...
>
> ...If they stole your rights
> And you're lost in the night
> When skies don't look bright
> My friend don't lose sight
> When you just cannot fight no more
> That's when I need you
> That's when I really need you
> That's when I need you to call me"

My story from the past year was to be told in words of contemporary secular music, as little music within the particular Christian tradition with which I am familiar speaks to me at any depth of feeling. Maybe this would resonate with other people, maybe it would not. I felt that folk were free to take from the whole what they found helpful and discard what they found otherwise.

Robin (my youngest brother) sang Psalm 139 to a setting, which he had composed. The psalm is meaningful to me, but hard. If God knew about Jamie, when he was growing in my womb – as I always believed – God knew too about Jennifer (and the fact that she could not survive the birth experience, because of her severe heart defect). God also knew (when I was in the womb) that I am probably carrying a gene that predisposes me towards cancer (for which confirmation, I am still awaiting genetic test results).

"O Lord, you have searched me and known me...
For it was you who formed my inward parts; you
knit me together in my mother's womb.
I praise you, for I am fearfully and wonderfully
made...
My frame was not hidden from you, when I was
being made in secret, intricately woven in the
depths of the earth.
Your eyes beheld my unformed substance.
In your book were written all the days that were
formed for me, when none of them as yet existed."
[Verses from Psalm 139: New Revised Standard
Version Bible]

ACT ONE – BREAKDOWN

★

I was VERY angry when active cancer was diagnosed for the second time. For a long time I was in a place where I had no desire to acknowledge God. The rock music of Meatloaf helped me to express that anger, particularly the track "Life is a Lemon" from the album "Bat out of Hell II – Back Into Hell" (1993):

"It's all or nothing and nothing's all I ever get
Every time I turn it on, I burn it up and burn it out
It's always something, there's always something going
wrong
That's the only guarantee, that's what this is all about

It's a never-ending attack
Everything's a lie and that's a fact
Life is a lemon and I want my money back!

What about love? It's defective, it's always breaking in
half
What about sex? It's defective, it's never built to really
last
What about your family? It's defective, all the batteries
are shot
What about your friends? They're defective, all the
parts are out of stock
What about hope? It's defective, it's corroded and

decayed
What about faith? It's defective, it's tattered and it's
frayed
What about your gods? They're defective, they forgot
the warranty
What about your town? It's defective, it's a dead end
street to me
What about your school? It's defective, it's a pack of
useless lies
What about your work? It's defective, it's a crock and
then you die
What about your childhood? It's defective, it's dead
and buried in the past
What about your future? It's defective, and you can
stuff it up your ass!"

Gradually, I recognized through my anger that, for many people, life never gave them even half a chance. It seemed trite to pull out that old chestnut, "there are always some people better off and there are always some worse off than you", but it remained true. Elie Wiesel (1981) and Primo Levi (1987) both experienced evil beyond our worst nightmares in Auschwitz. The genocide in recent times in Zimbabwe, as documented by Fergal Keane for BBC Television (2002), is beyond belief. All these, and the fact that my friend, Jose, was soon to be executed in Texas (or so we thought at the time) showed how hard life can be for so many people. Words from Bon Jovi's song "Hey God" (1995) seem to recognise this fact, so I played them next:

"She's a working single mom, like a
saint she don't complain
She never says a word, but she thinks that she's to
blame

Her son just got convicted, he blew
some cop away
She did her best to raise him, but the world got in the
way

Hey God – tell me what the hell is going on...
It keeps on getting harder hanging on
Hey God, there's nights you know I want to scream
These days you're even harder to believe
I know how busy you must be,
But Hey God... do you ever think about me?

I'd get down on my knees,
I'm going to try this thing your way
Seen a dying man too proud to beg
Spit on his own grave
Was he too proud to save?
Did you even know his name?
Are you the one to blame?
I got something to say... Hey God..."

ACT TWO: RECONCILIATION

★

There came a time when I began to connect with God again, though my understanding of God and God's nature has changed vastly in the course of these past years. One day, it felt as though the words of "Believe" by Ronan Keating (2000), were being spoken to me and God was saying that God still believed in me:

> "You said you could see no end
> The world and himself were all on your back
> I vowed to take your hand
> Show the world in a different light
> All that you've done
> You've got to believe
> In all of your dreams
> No matter what the world can throw at you
> You know you can believe
> Believe in me
> And after all
> I still believe in you."

Healing moments had come through the previous year's long, sunny summer, when I was recovering from my hysterectomy, such as the one experienced whilst lying on the bed listening to a short programme on Radio Four (Harvey, 28 June 2001) about the poem "Adlestrop" by Edward Thomas (one of the poets of the First World War). It tells of a moment captured in time, when

nothing actually happened, yet everything was happening and
something was caught of the essence of being alive:

> "Yes, I remember Adlestrop –
> The name, because one afternoon
> Of heat the express-train drew up there
> Unwontedly. It was late June.
>
> The steam hissed. Someone cleared his throat.
> No one left and no one came
> On the bare platform. What I saw
> Was Adlestrop – only the name,
>
> And willows, willow-herb and grass,
> And meadow-sweet and haycocks dry,
> No whit less still and lonely fair
> Than the high cloudlets in the sky.
>
> And for that minute a blackbird sang
> Close by, and round him, mistier,
> Farther and farther, all the birds
> Of Oxfordshire and Gloucestershire."
> (Collins, 1946 : 399)

ACT THREE: GRIEF

★

My experience during this period of my life was of grief following on after reconciliation to God and a certain acceptance of the fact of my illness; in other words, when I was getting better again, grief almost unexpectedly caught up with me. It entailed mourning for all that has been lost, for the things that can never be the same again. I acknowledged that I live now with controlled disease. I don't want that to be so, but it is. I wished that I could go back to the innocence I experienced when the world was all before me, when I had no expectation of dying. Yet I recognised that I can never regain such innocence, even if I live to be a very old lady.

R.S. Thomas' poem "Remembering", was written (I think) after his wife's death and speaks very much to me about this grief-full passing of time:

> "Love her now
> for her ecstasies,
> her willingness to oblige.
> There will come a time
> She will show her love for you in her cooking,
> Her sewing; in a bed made up
> for passionless sleeping.
>
> The wrinkles will come upon her

calm though her brow be
under time's blowing. Frost will visit
   her hair's midnight and not
thaw. Her eyes that were a fine day
   will cloud over
and rain down desultory
tears when, as she infers,
you are not looking. Your part then
will be to take her hand in your
   hand, proving to her
that if blind, it is not dumb.
(1996 : 78)

Many of the hits of Bruce Springsteen contain much in the way of nostalgia. This is especially true for me, as they take me back to my University days. In the last year of our shared accommodation on the edge of a common on the outskirts of Swansea, one of the guys always used to have his windows wide open. The curtains would be blowing outside and the music of Springsteen would blast across the yard!

"You and me, we were the pretenders,
We let it all slip away.
In the end what you don't surrender,
Well, the world just strips away..."
["Human Touch"]

"I got a job working construction for a Johnstown
company,
But lately, there ain't that much work on account of
the economy.
Now all them things that seemed so important
Well, mister, they vanished into the air.

Now I just act like I don't remember and Mary acts
like she don't care…"
["The River"]

"Just sitting back trying to recapture
A little of the glory…
But time slips away and leaves you with nothing,
mister,
But stories of glory days…"
["Glory Days"]

Verses from the Gospel of Saint John in the New Testament tell
of the way that Mary (a friend of Jesus) was met in the garden of
his tomb on Easter morning. These verses say to me, that our
grief becomes bearable, when we are met within it and called by
name:

"Mary stood weeping outside the tomb… she turned
around and saw Jesus standing there, but she did not
know that it was Jesus. Jesus said to her, 'Woman,
why are you weeping? Whom are you looking for?'
Supposing him to be the gardener, she said to him,
'Sir, if you have carried him away, tell me where you
have laid him, and I will take him away.' Jesus said to
her, 'Mary!' She turned and said to him in Hebrew,
'Rabbouni!' (which means Teacher).
(NRSV Bible : 109)

ACT FOUR: NEW COVENANT (NEW RELATIONSHIP)

★

By the time of this Rite of Passage, I had come to believe that there has to be a way forward in life, whilst recognizing our grief and all that has been lost to us. Kathy Keay's writings are particularly poignant to me, because she herself died at a young age as a result of breast cancer. After receiving a card from a friend, printed with the words, "We cannot direct the wind, but we can adjust our sails," I was able to include Keay's poem "Choice" in my liturgical drama:

> "Will you continue
> To exhaust yourself
> Battering yours wings
> Against immovable bars?
> Or will you learn
> To live
> Within the confines
> Of your prison
> And find to your surprise
> That you have
> The strength to sing
> Even there."
>   (1996 : 125)

It was followed by "Thank you for Loving Me", another track

from Bon Jovi's album "These Days" (1995), to say thank you to those who had helped and continued to help pull me through a difficult time in my life:

"It's hard for me to say the things I want to say some-
times
There's no-one here but you and me and a broken
old street light
Lock the doors and leave the world outside
All I've got to give to you is these fine words tonight

Thank you for loving me
For being my eyes when I couldn't see
For parting my lips when I couldn't breathe
Thank you for loving me...

You pick me up when I fall down
You ring the bell before they count me out
If I was crying you would comfort be
And you set out to rescue me..."

The service continued with set prayers from "A Wee Worship Book" of the Wild Goose Worship Group, belonging to the Iona Community in Scotland. I consider liturgical prayer to be very helpful, when you have no words to pray yourself and the particular set I found resonated in my mind with Jose's situation as he rapidly approached the date of his execution:

"Let us pray for those who may be born today...
The joy of God shine from your face and joy to all
who see you;
The shield of God surround your head, and angels
ever guard you.

May every season be good for you
And the Son of Mary give peace to you...

Let us pray for those who face death today...
May God provide for you all that is needed
For body, mind and soul as you face the final journey.
May Christ take your soul in his arms,
And bring you through the balancing time
To the dwelling place of peace and make it your
home for ever."
(1999 : 33)

We did sing three hymns as part of our liturgy, two of which Jeremy and I had sung at our wedding eighteen years previously. The closing hymn was a favourite Easter hymn of mine, written by John of Damascus, about 750 CE. Although Church structures have often left me feeling quite negative, I have valued being part of a chain of people through the centuries, who have tried to express their sense of God's presence in life by means of their Christian faith:

"The day of resurrection,
Earth, tell it out abroad!
The passover of gladness,
The passover of God!
From death to life eternal,
From earth unto the sky,
Our Christ has brought us over
With hymns of victory!"
("Hymns & Psalms" : 208)

However, I chose for the finale, the track "Brighter Days" from the album "Ronan" (2000):

"I've done a lot of living in my life
Chased my share of rainbows in the sky
Before I stopped to ask the question why
I've fallen out of love too may times

But now I see
The possibilities
Of how my life could be

From any other love I'd walk away
Love is temporary I would say
Now each night I find a reason to stay
With you there's always brighter days..."

Part Two

October 2003 – November 2004

"This above all – to refuse to be a victim"

[Margaret Atwood]

EMAIL TO IAN 4 OCTOBER 2003

★

I was glad to receive your letter and know how you are going on and I am glad that you have reached a place where you are accessing some strategic "tools" for your onward journey in life. I was going to tell you my feelings on the subject you raised, but isn't it risky to talk on the level of really telling other people what you think?! On the other hand, I don't think either of us minds if/when the other person doesn't agree with us. Neither do we assume that the other will agree with us. We seem to have reached a place, at least between ourselves, of knowing that it's the exchange of ideas that is so essential for personal growth.

So, I feel safe to say that it looks like you are 'suffering from' something similar to me. It took my friend Sarah to catch hold of it for me. It is the fact that we have both been on such enormous growing sprees in recent months/years that we have kind of left some of our former friends in a different place. They don't understand/can't relate to us, because we are not now the people they knew and they (for whatever reason) have not grown in the same way/have declined the growth process. We, on the other hand, have not had that option, because if we had refused the journey, we would have been dead by now – me, literally, you, "just" inside from the heaped up shit that is depression, which makes me think of the people attacked by the spectres in Pullman's "Subtle Knife". If you haven't read his trilogy, you must. They are supposed to be novels for teenagers, but by gum, is all I can say. I am sure that there must be a window between worlds at the bottom of our garden!

You will realise, I trust, from the speech marks I have put, that I don't think there is any "just" in being dead from depression. I only used the word – probably badly – to try and distinguish from the process of physical death, though I suppose this kind of dying is a stage on the way to the physical dying. Speaking for myself at the moment, I don't know what the future will hold. It is only possible in this scenario to live one day at a time. We have had a lot of added pressure, because I was worried about lumps under my arms again, but all points to chemo and radiotherapy damage. I have been to the hospital several times in recent weeks, so I must just now try and grasp hold of life and live it!!

What can I say, except affirm you in the journey you are trying so hard to make, validate you and wish you well in your job search? Sorry to have been so absent for so long, but you have been much in my thoughts!
Love Lesley X

EMAIL TO PETER, 6 OCTOBER 2003

★

After a scare in the last few weeks, my doctors have confirmed that I am (as people keep telling me I look) probably fitter than I have been for a number of years and both my GP and consultants say that I should not focus on the possibility of the cancer's return. However, Jeremy has not been well. In fact he has been quite poorly and has realised (with our GP's support) that he has probably been quite depressed for a long time, partly as a result of all the stress and strain he has been under in recent times due to my illness and treatment. He has always been able to work, but has not been able to do much else for quite a while, and as he is also permanently on the 2-10pm shift these days, I have been feeling a bit like a single parent in all the tasks I've had to do alongside my paid employment! But that is life for many people. He is getting steadily better now (though it will be a while yet before he has completely regained his equilibrium), so life is less fraught as he can cook a meal and make his own sandwiches for work again! The latter and the fact that I have had a lot of problems with my email have kept me fairly out of contact with the wider world and friends at a distance in recent weeks. Now Jamie has successfully logged me on to Hotmail.

It's coming up to two years (in November) since the night I took an evening airing, instead of the usual afternoon one, because you had called unexpectedly; and ended up being 'found' by an abandoned dog! Sophie is probably one of the best things that ever happened to me!!! Hope you are well.

All the Best,
From Lesley

EMAIL TO IAN, 14 OCTOBER 2003

★

Sorry about your sleeplessness and increasing age and infirmity!!
I am, of course, speaking as one who has to put her specs on first
in the morning and take them off last at night – so also increasingly aged and infirm!! The autumn colours are pretty amazing
here too – took Sophie for a long walk on Sunday – a free day
after two Sundays when I'd worked all day. Mum and Dad have
done us a good turn in 'selling' us mum's car at book price (they
don't need two, now she's retired). The power steering is unbelievable re my shoulder – what a difference it makes.

Don't start looking for what might go wrong in your life at the
moment! It is a dreadful temptation, which has always been just
round the corner for me – as soon as I think that life might be
getting ok, I get suspicious! What has happened in my shut
away memory to make me so mistrustful of life, because this
feeling comes from way before things like Jennifer's stillbirth
and my cancer? Nowadays, I think Jeremy and I both cope
better with the uncertainties of life, by admitting to them. It's
funny, it's another bit of wisdom that the Jesus guy got to before
me – he talked about having to let go of your life to be able to
live it.

I think I have aged one hundred years in the last months. Down
to a very low dose of antidepressants now, so life has a different
aspect feelings-wise – a better one.

Lots of love from Sophie, Flopsy, Mopsy, Cottontail, Charles and William (latter five are out late tonight – they didn't go out till late afternoon and I need to clean their hutches before I get them in) Baggy and Pepe send purrs!!

EMAIL TO IAN, 17 OCTOBER 2003

★

Thank you for your reflection. I printed it out and read it and dreamt about it (I'm doing a lot of dreaming these days). It helped me to see what is under my nose – the good friend I have in you, which I do appreciate. What I appreciate is being able to talk to you and know that you will not necessarily agree with me. In fact, you may disagree strongly, but that is OK. It is the ability to air ideas without prejudice or condemnation that is so helpful.

Me and two of my women friends are going on a poetry day tomorrow, between Ledbury and Ross on Wye – at some old house with lunch and tea thrown in all for £20 – am looking forward to it immensely. My shoulder has been playing up and it was sore before I went to bed last night. Suspect it's the result struggling with the mechanism of our new car lock – never bothered to lock the old one. No one would have pinched the old Skoda, but an increase in car crime in the town centre means I don't want our fairly new Fiesta nicked.

Love Lesley, Sophie, F, M, C, C & W, B & P

The animals need to be put out in the cold bright sunshine, but I know you get upset if they don't send you a few furry greetings!

LETTER TO JOSE
TUESDAY 21 OCTOBER 2003

★

Dear Jose, Here I am again at last! How are you? Hope that you got the money that we sent – it wasn't a lot, but I hope it was some help. C and J both gave me a little to send to you. C seems to be doing quite well after his surgery earlier in the summer. J keeps well and is doing well at her job of managing a charity shop in one of the local shopping centres. It's always pleasant to go into her shop – it is bright and welcoming. She works hard to achieve the targets that are set for her by her bosses. Making money via second hand clothing is big business these days (it's hard to believe the things that some people throw away). J works for a charity that raises money to ensure that older people live in suitable and helpful environments.

We are all going on reasonably well. Have I told you that Jeremy permanently works the 2-10pm shift these days? It means that I have to see to anything the children need in the week, so I don't always have a lot of time for anything else. For instance, Jamie is applying for University places at the moment (for next September). We went to look at a couple of the Universities that he is interested in. Liverpool (which is a two hundred mile round trip) had a mid-week open day, so I had to drive Jamie up there myself. Then on the Saturday, we went across to Nottingham (one hundred mile round trip), but Jeremy was able to come and share the driving that time. It is a big help to me that Mum and

Dad have let us have their second car and we can pay them for it in easy payments. So we have two very old cars parked out back, that we hope to sell for a little capital, but it won't be much! We had to take our second car off the road (when we were running two old ones) when my salary went down to half-time pay.

Jamie and I still go to the gym once a week (though we missed the week when we had all the travelling to do). He goes on all the equipment. I just go on the upright bike and the treadmill and do some stretching exercises and then sit and wait for him. I am SLOWLY building up. Last night, I rode 3 kilometres on the bike at level four of difficulty (easiest is one and goes up to about twelve) – it took me nine and a half minutes. Then I walked one kilometre on the treadmill. I do that at a speed of five kilometres an hour, on a very slight uphill gradient, as I find that easier. I am not aiming to lose weight (I am supposed to remain steady weight-wise from my doctors' point of view), but I am toning up.

When we got home I walked Sophie, though she doesn't like it at the moment, because of the fireworks, which are going off because of Diwali celebrations (Hindu festival). Then it will be Bonfire Night on 5 November. It is almost two years since we first had her, which is hard to believe. Don't know what I would do without her!

Katie is growing VERY fast. She is so tall now, will soon be past me. She has been saving her money like mad for a long time. We had a SMALL insurance come out last month, so we went halves with her and bought her the drum kit she has wanted for some time. She has had drum lessons for the last year at school and was getting worried because she couldn't practice at home and has her first exam in December. She is good. Now I have heard her play,

I see why she wants to practice. She has to keep so many rhythms going at once on the different drums. With the rest of the money she'd saved, we bought a new bike for her yesterday – traded her old one in. She could hardly ride her old one now with her long legs, and Jamie and she go riding Saturdays. Jamie borrows Jeremy's bike – Jeremy has lost a lot of weight and is getting fit riding to work each day. It is hard to believe how fast my children are growing up!

Did I tell you that Jeremy has not been well? He has been very depressed (now I am well, all the worry from when I was ill has been catching up on him). He has been on tablets for about two months now and he is gradually starting to feel better. That means I have a bit more time. I haven't been able to keep in touch with any of my friends, what with my work and keeping the house and family together while he was ill. I felt a bit like a single parent must feel, especially when he wasn't even feeling like he could pack his own sandwiches for work – fortunately, he has always been able to go to work. So things are improving round here.

Our friend in Dallas was saying she would like to see us again. I wonder if it might be possible later next year? We shall have to see. I would love to get back to Texas. Jeremy is right, we would never have come there in the first place if it hadn't been for you, so knowing you has broadened our horizons and made our world better! I know you will understand why I haven't written recently, but I wish that it was not so. I hope things are reasonable for you at the moment. I must go. It is time to go to another meeting, about some development work that we want to take place at one of my churches.

EMAIL TO IAN
WEDNESDAY 5 NOVEMBER 2003

★

I just fell through another door................

> *"One great discouragement to great souls in the Persuit of*
> *Felicity is the solitariness of the way that leadeth to her*
> *Temple. A man that studies Happiness must sit alone like*
> *a sparrow upon the House Top and like a Pelican in the*
> *Wilderness. And the reason is because all men Prais*
> *happiness and despise it: very few shall a man find in the*
> *way of Wisdom... Either he must go on alone, or go back*
> *for company. People are tickled with the Name of it, and*
> *som are persuaded to enterprise a little, but quickly draw*
> *back when they see the trouble yea cool of themselves*
> *without any Trouble. Those mysteries which while men are*
> *ignorant of it they would give all the Gold in the world for,*
> *I have seen when known to be despised. Not as if the*
> *Nature of Happiness is such that it needed a vail: but the*
> *nature of Men is such, that it is odious and ungratefull. For*
> *those things which are most glorious when most Naked, are*
> *by men when most Nakedly revealed most despised."*
> (Traherne: Centuries of Meditations 4.13)

I never knew Traherne before. A book about him was by my
bed. I 'came upon it' at a poetry day that I went to near Ledbury
a couple of Saturdays ago. I had not had chance to look at it. It

'accosted' me as I got out of bed this morning. I have always believed in books being for 'right times' to be read. The exclusive language and spellings come from the time. He was a man who was of a cheerful disposition and loved light, though his childhood had been difficult. He also appears to have been part of the subversive, rather than prevalent culture of the church. I found Traherne's words, just as the words of The Jam had been running through my mind "Going Underground...." and I had begun to realise that any part I have to play in God's kingdom is going to be subversive and small from now on, but it is in the small tasks, the seed sowing, that growth begins. My role will also perhaps be kind of "incognito", as just another person in another house living an ordinary life.

The true irony in all the pain for me is the fact that, it is the very thing that keeps me alive that some people seem to most dislike about me! I cannot be other than a fighting, life-challenging person. And for the first time ever, I am allowing the life spirit in me to be creative, instead of drugging it up with depression and medication. But the truth is that the structures that rule the world want us to be drugged... Arghhh!!!!!! I just fell into "The Matrix", which we saw again on TV the other day and I know how much you love Neo!!!

Lesley X

And Sophie, Flopsy, Mopsy, Cottontail XXXX

EMAIL TO IAN LAST SUNDAY IN NOVEMBER (ADVENT SUNDAY) 2003

★

Do you realise that you used the word 'enjoy' twice in that last mail? Things must be looking up, which is good. Had my biopsy result Friday – it is the cancer back. I see my oncologist Wednesday, when we'll see what to do. We should also have the result of my bone scan then. Last week was stressful with the biopsy and scan. I have been feeling REALLY tired this weekend as a result. Found my service tonight really physically tiring.

Everyone is saying, "It's so lovely to see you looking so well these days!" Grr! Think I told you my chest X-ray was clear. Booked for an ultrasound on my stomach cavity. I anticipate that will also be OK, but couldn't cross my heart and say I feel the same way about my bone scan, particularly in relation to my left shoulder. Think about me Wednesday, 3pm our time, please. At least there are several treatments that I haven't yet had, so I don't intend to turn up my toes quite yet, but I'm not ecstatic about the idea of more chemo.

Cheers,
Lesley X

EMAIL TO ALISON, 6 DECEMBER 2003

★

Dear Alison – This is to wish you a Happy Birthday, as I rather think you won't get your card till Monday. Thank you for my birthday card and please forgive the slowness of getting in touch by email. Life just seems to slip away these days! We will have been in our house a year on the twenty-third of this month, which means you must have been moved into yours a lot longer. Something has gone wrong with our system, as neither of us has seen the other's new house and we don't usually go years at a stretch without seeing each other! I guess it's just to do with our conflicting work patterns, but perhaps we can get something pencilled in for the New Year?!

How was OFSTED? I guess it's past, looking at the date of your note. Hopefully, all was OK for you, and most of all, I hope that your sleeping patterns are improving. You say you need news from beyond school, but I am not sure the news I have to tell is the sort that you need just now.

Your birthday is (unfortunately) also the anniversary of my original cancer diagnosis. Seven years ago today. Seven years living with a controlled disease, which I didn't realise in the beginning and probably couldn't have coped with then. But you get used to these things. The hospital has been keeping an eye on me over recent weeks/months, as I wasn't happy about under my left arm (again). They couldn't find anything and blood tests didn't reveal anything; but to cut a long story short (a story which I tend not to tell people – I feel quite differently about how I deal with this these days and mostly don't want to tell people on a day-to-day level – except close friends, because most people don't understand about living with controlled disease and the "C" word just makes them upset or worried)...

.... to cut a long story short, the cancer is active again (with tumours under my arm and in the skin where my left breast was), though my chest X-ray (for my lungs) and my bone scan were clear. I have an ultrasound scan next week to look at my stomach cavity, but I reckon that'll be ok. If it was in my liver, I don't think I would be as well overall as I am.

My left arm is severely swollen because of the tumours under my arm, which are blocking the drainage of my lymph system. This swelling (lymphodema) is restricting my movement and causing some discomfort, so it's time to treat the disease. They don't rush straight in for someone like me, as it's quality of life we're talking about, and treatment would no doubt be effective (again), but would make me ill again, no doubt. The good news last Wednesday was that we are going to try a new hormone treatment first (rather than wading straight in again with chemotherapy). Tamoxifen and Arimidex are both hormone therapies, which stopped working for me a couple of years ago now, but both were effective initially. So I'm trying a hormone therapy from a different family (Megace – progesterone based) to see if it will have any effect. I go back to see the consultant on something like 5 January, by which time they'll have my ultra-sound result, and we may be on the way to getting a clue as to whether Megace will have any effect (though the blurb says it takes about two months to work). I know Arimidex shrunk the tumour that was in my neck two years ago quite quickly, so I'm hopeful. Anyway, it means I won't be ill for Xmas. If this doesn't work, or if there was cancer in my liver (but I'm sure there's not), it would automatically be chemo – one of the two drugs based on the yew, which are supposed to be very good.

Overall, I am well; I just have active cancer (again!). Mind you, when I see that there is a risk of blood clot from this new drug (which the blurb – to cover the drug company – does warn can occasionally be fatal), I do feel a bit like I am playing roulette with my life. Which button to press today? Shall we choose death by clotting, poisoning (chemo) or cancer growth? I don't write to upset you. This is my life and, overall, the irony is that I am enjoying it these days. The fraught things at work, I can avoid. There are a couple of good projects underway to focus on till I hand over to the next person, though in the work context, the most frustrating thing about this disease is the way that it means I lose choices in life.

On the other hand, I love our house and really appreciate the time I get to spend with the kids, who both got good reviews in parent evenings (I have to do all the family things as Jeremy is permanently on 2-10pm these days). Jamie has had conditional offers from all the universities he has applied for (re Accounting) so far, except Liverpool. They are Nottingham Trent, Leeds, Sheffield Hallam, Manchester Metropolitan & Wolverhampton. Liverpool & Nottingham Trent are favourite for his course. Sadly, broke up with his girlfriend earlier this term, after well over a year of relationship. It knocked him off course for a while, but he seems to be back on target and one advantage is we've done some things together as a family again, which we appreciate, as we know that we will miss him when he goes off to university.

Katie is almost as tall as me (about half an inch to go). Thirteen now. Very high grades at parent evening. Drum kit installed in room beside me – she has her first drum exam before the end of term. Growing pains in her legs again today – she is a bit prone to them. She's about to play her drums to Jamie and his friend, who both play guitar. Jamie has been practising a lot and is getting good. We bought him an acoustic guitar when we bought Katie's drum kit. He reckons he can take an acoustic to university more easily than his electric guitar.

Jamie keeps trying for part-time jobs, no luck so far, but one hopeful one in the pipeline at the moment – he needs the cash! Jeremy is improving depression-wise, though he got a bit knocked back in the last week or two worrying about me. You knew he'd been quite poorly didn't you? Managed to keep going to work, but that was about all at one point. Well on the mend, though occasionally I still have to do things I shouldn't – like march him to the barber's this morning. Part of the depression is not being able to take adequate care of himself – on days like today, I say I have three children! Though that was just a blip this morning. The days of me having to do his lunchbox and keep an eye on him like that are mainly past, thank goodness, and he can help in the house again. I am amazed retrospectively how much he has done here to make this such a nice home, when I consider how poorly he must have been for such a long time, without me picking up on it. Bet you wish I hadn't got back in touch! Must stop! Drums about to deafen me!

Love Lesley X

EMAIL TO IAN, 5 JANUARY 2004

★

Hi – Thank you for your New Year greetings. Hope 2004 turns out to be what you would like it to be. Sorry not to have been in touch. I think I am turning into a non-communicating creature. I find I have less I want to say to anyone about anything. I don't know if it is age, or to do with getting my head round what I live with.

We had a restful holiday period. Some days with Mum and Dad and some time alone at home, when we were able to do some blitzy kind of jobs, like clearing the cellar and the top of the stairs. We can now shut our bedroom door for the first time since we moved in! I have had the heavy fluey cold that a lot of folk have had. It has lasted over a fortnight and has left me feeling pretty rough. Days like today, I'm glad I'm only half-time, because I'll be able to spread my hours out through the week and just potter gently though.

It makes me wonder what will happen later in the year, as (realistically) what other jobs could I work the hours in the shapes that suit me? There are a lot of things to wait and see with. If they offer me a viable retirement package, maybe I should take that? I don't know. It'll partly depend what they say at the hospital next week. These hormone tablets appear to be working. Certainly have stopped the tumours from growing. I am getting movement back in my arm and shoulder – is it any wonder my immune system is struggling? Colds and cancer are a lot to throw at it all at once, but it seems to battle nobly on.

I have worked through a lot in these seven years. I feel quite realistic about where I am re my cancer. I live with it, but I don't want to dwell on it, and don't really want to talk about it to folk any more. Not because I'm in denial. I know quite well what I live with, but most people don't yet understand the concept of controlled disease – certainly not CANCER – and I don't want their pity or their upset. I just want to find the best way to live through all this. And mostly (apart from now and this 'flu' thing), I am pretty well.

I am glad that I can see the end of this job. I need a change – whatever the change may be. I have permission to be Without Appointment. So I think that will be the end of my preaching – at least for the time being. It is getting increasingly hard. How did I do it before? Well I always had a lot to say!!! Now I don't! The good things are being able to root myself in one place (no threat of having to move on again), and the slight hint of spring in the air. How did you get on assisting or whatever in worship again? Are you any clearer about your way forward? I am sorry to have been a bit of an absent friend in recent weeks, but I think I have been a bit absent from everyone.

Love from us all – and all the menagerie X

EMAIL TO IAN 16 JANUARY 2004

★

The cold sounds cold! Huddling round a wood fire (with thoughts of the draughts whistling round behind you) sounds yeuk! Sorry about the situation at work – life, eh?! Maybe you need some stimulation to help overcome the tiredness. What would you like to do?! (Maybe you shouldn't answer that question!)

Well, now we know that I have permission to go "Without Appointment", there is a noticeable lack of anyone taking any interest in seeing how I am. It's the old syndrome, witnessed many times through my career – the person who doesn't fit in, somehow just gets sidelined. Never mind, except when I remind myself that the reason most of everything has happened in my life recently (in terms of growth and change as a person) is just because I've been getting my head round living with cancer. A mere nothing. So inconsiderate of me. But I won't push that sentiment, because I don't want to be known as/for the disease, but it is a consideration!

Pardon me for saying this, but I suspect that living with disability (in my case disease) is as much a "please, must we acknowledge/ talk about it?!" situation for the Church as acknowledging these persistently inconsiderate women and gay people, who insist on muddying the edges of life. Wouldn't life be simpler, if everything could be kept orderly and tidy for the Church, to be "sorted out" by the people (previously always men, but nowadays including some women) with the answers and the grace to be obliging and work the system?! The people that is, who haven't yet nose-dived to the reality that, basically, life sucks!

I do accept that I probably won't know till I almost finish here what is next, because that appears to be the nature of the faith life, which is a huge joke, because the Church that professes to live by that substance usually can't, because it is so tied into the forward planning, in which those of us with no fixed future can no longer participate. Again, so inconsiderate of me not to want to commit in the structures to what I might do a year ahead! Hello!! What I might want to do is be alive!! If I am (and only when I know that I am) I might offer to do something for you. But it will be then, not now in advance!

Does any of this ranting make any sense to you? See, you must have suspected that what I really needed was a good rant! Maybe what has started this one is the fact that I sometimes feel invisible to other people these days (though I suppose there's really no change there, as there are lots of situations in life where being a woman renders me invisible anyway). Therefore, in case you might be suffering from the same inability to see (though in your case, it would be most likely due to extreme cold and lack of blood to the head), just in case you are confused about the invisible blot on the horizon that is sending you this email, could I point out that it is me... that I *do* exist, and that (far from finding me an inconvenience for mucking up life by having cancer), God seems (at times) quite apologetic about it all and definitely sympathetic. Even going so far as to suggest, there might be ways through this mess and that if it comes to the crunch eventually (i.e. death) well, I won't be on my own. Meanwhile, God is doing a pretty good job of sorting out the particular mess that was made cancer-wise when God set creation going, by getting all these creative men and women to find ways of treating the 'damned' disease – pardon my 'French'!

My consultant was pleased at the hospital on Wednesday. Megace appears to be working, though hormone therapy tends to show whether or not it'll be effective long-term, rather than in the short-term. But the six weeks I've been on it has provided relief from the lymphodema (fluid retention) in my arm. I have more movement again and have been able to do things round the house over the Xmas period, like clear the cellar with Jeremy, which I couldn't have managed previously. Also not waking up in the night in pain and able to sleep in quite a variety of positions again, whereas I'd been reduced to about one. Megace can have a side effect of fluid retention/breathlessness; so he's prescribed me a mild diuretic, as when I get dressed or walk and talk simultaneously I can sound like a tramp steamer in high seas; but (hey) life is a trade off when you get to the long-term stage of drug therapy that I'm at. What's a bit of breathlessness, compared to controlling cancer in a way that is simultaneously poisoning your entire system, like chemo does?! You will soon be as pissed off by this cancer lark as some people round here seem to be!!! Hey, I only have to live with it in my body – sorry for offending your sensibilities!!!!!

Actually, apart from this jolly rant, I am at such a different stage than I have ever been in the seven years that this has been going on. I accept my condition in life now, in a way that I would never have before. That doesn't mean I 'put up with' the cancer – I suspect that that way lies certain death. But I know that this is my life – living with disease and combating it. Not knowing what the outcome will be, but being quite realistic about the disability.

Meanwhile, I try and get on with life. Have to fetch Jamie from a gig in the city at midnight. Then take him to work for 8.30am in the morning. Jeremy has just come in from work, is eating his supper, before going to work, as he is on 6am – 2pm tomorrow. Has to work Saturdays now, which helps financially. Means I am quite busy family/home wise, when not working. Been glad of a quiet week this week, as don't think I've quite left behind the fluey cold bug I had consistently over the Xmas period. Probably haven't done my hours, but then I did over the number last week and next week looks like it will be over-time as well. Part-time makes life a lot more flexible.

Katie is in bed. Time to go and leave you in peace. Hope you are OK. The rabbits love it now the cellar is cleared out. They get to race around inside in this inclement weather. Flopsy has been burrowing through the floor, removing the bricks and discovering the earth underneath! Sophie sends woofs. Baggy and Pepe send "miaows".

Lesley X

EMAIL TO IAN 25 JANUARY

★

Thanks for that poem. I've printed it off, because I will have to read it aloud to get the feel of it properly. Have been meaning to send you this for a few days. You know that R.S. Thomas is my very favourite poet?! Well, I got out the collection "No Truce With The Furies" the other day – one of his last collections (I think I have them all from the later years) and discovered this one – so much where I am at these days. We have had computer problems again – but one new hard drive and one purchase of Windows XP later – here we are again! Every time I think that I might have just a little spare cash this month, there – it's gone!

> The relation between us was
> silence; that and the feeling
> of each one being watched
> by the other: I by an
> enormous pupil in a blank
> face, he by one in a million
> wanderers in the darkness
> that was never a long way off
> from his presence.

> It had begun
> by my talking all of the time
> repeating the worn formulae
> of the churches in the belief

that was prayer. Why does silence
suggest disapproval? The prattling
ceased, not suddenly but,
as flowers die off in a frost
my requests thinned. I contented
myself I was answering
his deafness with dumbness. My tongue
lolled, clapper of a disused
bell that would never again
pound on him.

What are the emotions
of God? There was no admiring
of my restraint, no suggestion even
of a recompense for my patience.
If he had allowed himself but one
word: his name, for instance, spoken
ever so obliquely; my own that,
for all his majesty, acknowledged
my existence.

And yet there were creatures
around me with their ears
pricked; figures on ancient cathedrals,
the denizens of art, with their rapt,
innocent faces and heads on one side
as though they were listening. Ah, but to whom?
(1995 : 83)

LETTER TO VIOLET, 23 FEBRUARY 2004

★

Nice to hear from you. Thank you for your last letter and kind
good wishes. The weather is very variable at the moment isn't it?!
Very cold today, but bright. Snowdrops and daffodils in the park
when I took Sophie at 8.30am this morning. And squirrels –
which are, of course, the most important thing as far as Sophie is
concerned! Jamie works from 8.30am–2pm on Saturdays and
Sundays in another part of the city. We take him and he makes
his own way home, though today I am picking him up and we
are going into Birmingham to browse for an hour of two. I have
built an early morning routine around taking him to work on
Saturdays. Walk the dog on the way home at East Park (about a
mile around the perimeter). Into Lidl for the shopping about five
to nine when it's empty! Great! Then, anything I can't get there
(it's great, price wise) from Morrisons or Kwik Save. Home by
10.30am to snooze on the settee before putting the shopping
away!!

Saturday evening – Got a few minutes before going to watch
"The Regency House Party" on TV and then an early night. I
am quite tired today. My mother-in-law is in hospital (South
Wales). We had a weekend with friends in London last weekend
and came back via Newport to see Jeremy's Mum in hospital and
then went and had a cup of tea with his Dad before coming
home. I keep half term fairly free because of the kids, whom I
abandoned and went back to South Wales Tuesday morning till

Thursday night. So we have had a few things on our plate – with future uncertainties and some family worries. I feel things will work out in the end.

My main issue is, of course, living with controlled disease. Lumps started again under my arm and in the skin of the chest wall on the left side last autumn. All tests re other vital organs, etc remain clear, so I am trying a hormone therapy (new one called Megace). As long as it is doing something, it puts off chemo, which would be the next thing. It's about four months off two years since I last finished chemo, so I have done well to go so long without any.

I have moved a long way along the road of living with this situation and I accept it these days. Mostly, I am OK about it, though it brings some hard things. Accepting it doesn't mean giving in to it – I wouldn't still be alive if that were the case – but it makes life much more manageable to have moved through the bitter anger and grief that the initial stages of such a serious illness can bring with it; and I genuinely believe that God supports me through all this (though some people don't necessarily). Sometimes I get a bit caustic in my thoughts about other people's behaviour towards me in this situation, but the feelings don't last. I haven't got the time, energy, nor the inclination to be bitter. Mostly, a bit of irony and a chance to laugh help to relieve the negative feelings. Bet you wish you hadn't asked how things arc!!

It is the managing of the condition that makes the next stage of my life a little more uncertain. Once September is here and things have changed and I know which of the options I am pursuing, I am going to be living with, I think there will be an enormous sense of relief. Also I have an excellent relationship with the hospital. I was supposed to go back for another check up after two months, but I just rang this week and got an appointment next week, because I want someone who knows what they are looking at to check me over. They always fit me in if I have any queries. Once, when I was very worried, it was the same day that I rang. They know that patient participation makes the management of the disease much more successful. Anyway, enough of me. Hope all went well for your visit to Nottingham. I understand that a pacemaker can give quite a new lease of life. Do tell me the date of your seventieth, so that I can send a card to help you celebrate. Jamie is eighteen on 25 March, which is Lady Day! Incidentally, Jennifer would have been seventeen today.

Lesley

EMAIL TO CHRIS, 2 MARCH 2004

★

Sorry to hear that things have been a bit tough going, but it sounds like you dealt with the situation, instead of burying your head in the sand or going into denial or making excuses. In my experience (for what it is worth) people generally respond to honesty and attempts to be genuine with them. At the end of the day, they recognise (if we don't try and deny it) that we are all human and can make mistakes. And hey, life's like that, we make mistakes, we pull ourselves up by the bootstraps and we plough on. The damage to our self-esteem becomes a learning experience, if we let it and it's true that all things pass – this hard bit will pass and things will feel better, and then there might be some more hard bits, but they too will pass. I bought and read the novel "Damage" years ago (declined to watch the film later, because I thought it would be too sexually explicit for my visual taste), because of the quotation on the cover of the book. I recognized its truth then, and its truth remains, "Damaged people are dangerous – they know they can survive". Once you've survived one hard bit of life, you know you can get through the next. It doesn't mean things become less painful, it just means that you know you can get through them. Which makes you dangerous to other people sometimes, because they realise that they haven't got ultimate power over you.

Incidentally, we've had a couple of clear bits of the jigsaw this week. Retirement sounds the best option, so I will have a rest from 'minister-like' things from the end of August and clear my head.

Wednesdays I take my friend to painting classes – painting and computing are two of the things that are making me realise I can do things in life other than work and, that I am capable of learning new skills! But I have to be back by 4.15pm now that Katie has a paper round (her papers are delivered to the house and she can't always be back from school in time to receive them). So if you were to come here for about 4.15pm, that would be ok, otherwise we will have to renegotiate.

When I walked Sophie today, the sun at the top of the hill was brilliant in the frost – above a world in darkness. Yes, it is in so many ways, but that is too simplistic, when you consider the brightness…
    Lesley

EMAIL TO PAT, 5 MARCH 2004

★

Hi Pat – Hope David is doing OK. We have had a good think and a chat this end, and regretfully feel that if the pub doesn't work out on 14th, we will have to decline joining you at a later date, so it will be four less if you have to rebook the pub. Suggest you don't tell Dinah (my mother in law) that, because I don't want to put pressure on her – if she's not fit enough to go out on 14th, she's not fit enough and that's fair enough.

Sorry to be unhelpful, but **I** am my priority at the moment. My consultant and I are keeping an eye on the tumours under my left arm – it may yet be chemo, though I do think the Megace has had some beneficial effect and we're giving it a month longer, as it is slow working. I suspect it is not going to have the hoped for long-term effect of getting me back into remission. All of which is a pain in the bum, because as you know I am fairly fit and well at the moment, but chemo tends to make me feel 'off'. Hope the dogs are OK. I am just about to go and get rabbits and guinea pigs in for the night. They are out late, because Jamie and I finally got our act together and started back at the gym this evening. Jeremy should be home soon. Usually finishes at 9.30pm on a Friday.

Love Lesley.

EMAIL TO NEIL, 21 MAY 2004

★

Was cleaning computer table yesterday and found your Xmas card buried! Can't determine whether Jeremy has your new email, or when he last mailed you, so I thought I'd update you with his email address and leave it to you both from there! You will see he has had cause to be a little preoccupied!

His Mum has not been well since Xmas. She was in hospital once and came home, and then (to cut a long story short) it ended up with both his Mum and Dad in hospital. Taff was admitted on the Monday and I went to get Dinah admitted on the Thursday of the same week. That was 1 April. Taff came home with help about three weeks ago. Dinah got home this Monday, with a lot of help laid on. Her underlying condition is heart failure, so she won't recover to her previous state of health. She is better than she was (could have died), but Jeremy is adjusting to the reality of his parents' age (both in their 80s). It's a fair way to South Wales and Jeremy has the kind of job where you don't get paid if you don't work.

Meanwhile, I am off work at the moment, half way through another course of chemotherapy. It is doing what we want it to – knocking back the cancer, which has recurred under my left arm, but it is also making me feel a bit rough. Fortunately, so far, I have never had cancer anywhere to make me ill (vital organs, etc) and most people wouldn't know when I was dealing with it in an active stage by looking at me; but the treatment is always a big decision to undertake, because that does make me ill. I had to bite the bullet this time, because the tumours under my arm were causing lymphodema (fluid retention), which was getting painful and restricting movement and making driving difficult, for instance. After three doses of the drug (Taxol, this time) my arm is rapidly returning to its previous size and shape, so the treatment is obviously working, as the tumours that were blocking my system have obviously shrunk back.

So you can see that Jeremy has had a lot on his plate and tends to be a bit preoccupied from time to time! He is relaxing at the moment by building a glider. One advantage of being permanently on 2-10pm shift is that he can have a lie-in in the morning and potter a bit. It is helping him to get his head around all that is going on. I think he feels a bit better now his parents are both home and he can see my treatment is working.

Good news things – Jamie's last day at school today, before study leave for 'A' levels. Hopefully, he'll be off to Nottingham in the autumn to read Accounting. Very long hair now – well into 'piercings' now he's eighteen (partly because he's into heavy metal music). I'm going to miss him when he goes – it's nice having him around, but it's time for him to spread his wings. He's self-taught, but now pretty good and pretty fast playing on his guitar. Katie passed her Grade One Drum exam with Distinction. Currently beavering away at Grade Three. Seems well settled these days at St. Peter's. Glad we opted to stay in the area for the kids' benefit as much as anything. Katie gets on well with her Dad and they go on bike rides together. Well, I must stop now and do Jeremy a bit of lunch and do his lunch box. Weather grey and rainy. Hope life is OK with you.
All the Best, from Lesley.

LETTER TO ANN, 21 MAY 2004

★

I was sorry to receive your letter with news of L's death. This must be a hard time for you and your family. Thank you for sending me the order of service. I am sure that it must have been a comfort to you that L's body was able to rest for a night beside his choir stall, where he spent many happy times. It was good to see that D was able to read for his father. "Immortal, invisible" has always been a hymn whose words have held a lot of meaning for me – we used to sing it at school, so I know it by heart, but it has become richer over the years.

It cannot have been easy for any of you to watch L over recent months and know that you were not able to relieve him of the disease with which he was inflicted. I suspect that, because of the debilitating nature of Motor Neurone Disease and the amount of time with which L had to deal with it, that it is not really surprising that he did not come to terms with what was happening to him. I am afraid that life can be hard and when we find ourselves in bodies that no longer function as we are used to them doing, there is a kind of perplexity about the fact that "I am still in here and yet things are no longer as they were and can no longer be so again". That is very hard to take on board for ourselves, let alone share with others – and maybe we don't want to upset those nearest and dearest to us by such thoughts anyway. I have thought of L quite a lot and trust that the perplexity, and the grief and loss is now over for him; and that he is (as you say) at rest. I do have a strong underlying feeling that when the time comes for us to die, we are given the necessary comfort and strength to undergo the experience.

It's no good, I have a cat, who wants to sit on my knee, but I can't have him on here and type at the same time. I don't want claw marks in my legs, as I had another dose of chemotherapy this week – which is one of the reasons I would ask that you forgive the formality of print – it is easier to type than write at the moment. I think you know that I live with controlled breast cancer. At the end of March, I decide to "bite the bullet" and sign for another course of chemotherapy – it is always a big decision, as it is the treatment that makes me feel unwell. I am taking a course of Taxol (one dose every three weeks – six doses in all – infused in hospital during the course of an afternoon). The treatment seems to be having the desired effect and my consultant says I am already in partial remission, so I am hoping to achieve remission by the end of the course. It is however unlikely that I will ever be told that I am free of this disease, which is why I know a little of what it is like to be inside a body that no longer does what it once did, and will not be able to do some things again.

I have lived with this a long time now, and seem to have come through to a stage of acceptance about what I live with. That does not mean I give into it, but it does mean I use my energies to try and deal with it (the effects of the treatment and so on), instead of protesting and railing against God, the universe and everything. But I am not as disabled as L was (my disease has, so far, not been as vicious to me as his was to him), which is why I thought of him a lot. Cat has returned! Time to turn our thoughts to happier things!

Good things include the house. It was definitely the right

decision to settle here like this. It feels good to have a base and a rootedness for the children. We are steadily turning it into the kind of home we want it to be. Kitchen finally completed before my treatment began, all bar some tiling, which Jeremy is doing a bit at a time. Jamie's last day of school today, before breaking for study leave for his 'A' levels. All being well, he will be off to Nottingham to study Accounting in the autumn. I must get his grant forms out and start filling them out. Had a very late get-up this morning, so may be able to at least dig them out this afternoon, if not do anything about filling them out. I shall miss him a lot when he leaves, but it is time for him to spread his wings.

Katie at thirteen and a half is a teenager and we sometimes have related mother/daughter conflicts, but she seems to be doing OK at school and passed her first Drum exam with Distinction. We are proud of both the children and how well they have coped over the years with some of the abnormalities of our life style.

I am glad to be signed off work and I shall not be returning. The consultants who advise the Medical Committee to the Methodist Council are recommending that I be allowed to retire from the end of August. It has all to be finalised, but we knew it was the right direction in which to head, once we realised that it was a financially viable option. I need time for me and the family – no longer wish to juggle living with this condition and work. But once I am fit again after this course of treatment, I am looking forward to finding some things to do locally at my own pace – maybe popping into one of the schools to hear children read for instance. Nothing too demanding, but something a bit useful, to give a bit of structure to my week.

In amongst everything, Jeremy has had both his parents in

hospital at once in South Wales. They now need a lot of help at home. We are hoping to pop and see them during Whit week, but are going to my Mum's (near Wigan) because we both need a bit of a break first. Anyway, we are feeling better now that both his parents are home and my treatment is proving effective. Time to sign off. You will have had enough of my concerns. Thinking of you in the days ahead as you adjust to life without L – that is not an easy task that lies ahead of you. I am glad that you have such good support from your family to help you through this time.

Lesley

EMAIL TO DAVID, 27 MAY 2004

★

I have a lot of thinking time at the moment and although we haven't contacted your parents since Sunday, we have thought a lot about both of them and both of you. Actually haven't been well enough to ring them, as I had a bad night Monday and wasn't well Tuesday. Better again now. Some unpleasant side effects re last week's dose of chemo to do with nerve endings, optical nerves and hallucinations, amongst other things. Fortunately saw my doctors this week (as we'll be at Mum's next week), so was able to talk it all through with them and know which are likely to be passing side effects and what I should watch out for, that would be more serious and would need a dose adjustment.

Jeremy been doing lots of supporting and talking me through it, so also forgot to ring my Mum on her birthday (Tuesday), but doctors very pleased (would say excited) about efficacy of my drug and say I am on my way to remission, so we just have to grit our teeth and get on with it. Jeremy saw doctor today, who has given him two more months tablets − different kind with bit lower dose. Think Dr will probably let Jeremy stay on them till my treatment is finished, but he (Jeremy) is obviously feeling better, because he can see vast improvement in situation on my left chest wall.

So things are going OK − going to Mum's Sunday evening −

both need the break. It shouldn't make any difference sitting in the car to resting at home by that stage of this treatment cycle (halfway through the whole programme now). Hope Pat is OK. Let us know how things are going at number 59, please.

Lesley

EMAIL TO IAN, 7 JUNE 2004

★

Thank you for that word of affirmation! I also appreciate our friendship and conversations. Just found your two mails. My first chance to check since coming back from Mum's last Friday, as I 'crashed' a bit Saturday and then Sunday was a day trip to South Wales to see in-laws. Went for support for Jeremy, but can't really worry about them, as I have another dose of the 'nasty' tomorrow. It's as Yazoo sang, just as I feel better, "I get knocked down, but I get up again..."!

Trust your instincts. You can't know in advance how relationships will turn out. Sometimes they mess up – is that a reason not to relate or blame yourself?! I remember Simon and Garfunkel singing, "I am a rock, I am an island... and a rock feels no pain and an island never cries." We can't choose that way, surely? We plough on. Life is hard a lot, but the good bits make us hang on. What is it that Bruce Springsteen says in "Human Touch"?

> "That feeling of safety you prize, well it comes with a hard hard price. You can't shut off the risk and the pain without losing the love that remains. We're all riders on this train. So you been broken and you been hurt. Show me somebody who ain't. Yeah I know I ain't nobody's bargain, but hell a little touch up and a little paint..." (1995)

If you can continue to cope with an old crock, who needs more than a "touch up and a little paint" (I am still in here somewhere, honest, in this messed-up body, that is!) I can give you a bit of backup, albeit long-distance, when the risk taking, fear facing is too painful. On the other hand, sometimes we have to cut our losses... start again, recognizing it was never *all* our fault. It always takes two sides to make or break relationship.

Just printed off your other mail – think I will go to hospital tomorrow clutching that piece of Tennyson's "Ulysses" which you sent:

> "We are not now that strength which in old days
> Moved earth and heaven; that which we are, we are;
> Made weak by time and fate, but strong in will
> To strive, to seek, to find, and not to yield."
> (Collins, 1946 : 277)

Thank you for that – it is most timely and energizing. Need to dig out R.S. Thomas again – think I understand his "bone" references since my hallucinating of a week or so ago! Time to get in animals, feed Jeremy some supper... very hot here. Sophie, being black and white, having trouble coping.

Love Lesley X

EMAIL TO PAT, WEEK OF 8 JUNE 2004

★

Dear Pat – We were glad to see you – sorry to have caught you at a bad time. I am tired today, after treatment Tuesday. It is a huge adjustment to take on board the fact, that life can never be the same again. I have been on that pathway for seven and a half years now. I should think that Dinah has a lot to cope with at the moment, trying to deal with loss and impending mortality. It might help her to be able to talk about these kinds of issues with someone like a counsellor, or independent visitor, but I can't imagine that she would ever tackle them with a family member. Please try not to get too overwrought about it all. I think you both do a great job of support and David seems to have his finger on the pulse re keeping in contact with carers.

I am using my energy to try and live a bit longer yet! I should manage a bit further – one of the doctors at the hospital says I've "beaten the bookies"! If it helps you to cope with an argumentative sister-in-law, just remember that I wouldn't still be here if I hadn't got my particular attitude to life (much as it sometimes winds other people up!), as well as an amazingly supportive and caring husband (for whom I am genuinely thankful to Dinah and Taff) and people who will help me, when I need help, not to mention a first-class cancer centre near by. Enough! Sophie and I (and maybe Baggy Cat) are off to bed for the afternoon!

Love Lesley X

EMAIL TO NEIL, 18 JUNE 2004

★

Good to hear from you again. Thought I'd dash off a few replies on this machine, before going for a sleep! Managed to deliver Jamie's grant application forms to the Civic Centre this morning and did a short tutorial with someone I'm trying to see through a course on Worship and Preaching, before I finally "parachute" out of here! Having also cooked Jeremy's lunch and packed his lunch-box, what I have achieved (in current terms) is mega for one day, but I am about to fall asleep as a result!

R is obviously well independent these days, but then it is eight years since we left – hard to believe! Didn't know your Mum had died – sorry about Alzheimer's – it is a cruel disease. My Mum retired from ministry last summer – she is chirpy as a chicken and really enjoying her freedom (she was sixty-six this May – Dad a year older). Jeremy's Mum has been worrying us all, as she cancelled her complete care package (and his Dad's!). But this has been my tired week in my treatment schedule (lots of rest Mon/Tues/Weds), so I haven't been in contact with them – think she has consented to sort out a private cleaner, but when my energy levels are this low, I leave everyone to their own devices.

Sorry to know J was feeling low at your time of mailing – hope that she can keep working when she feels that way. I think when you live with particular physical conditions, you grow less and less willing to speak about them on a daily basis. The people who know you best know, and the rest don't need to know. I was very angry about my disease in the beginning – very angry with God that cancer existed at all. I am in a different place with regards to the disease and my thoughts about God these days. For myself, I have reached an acceptance that this is the way my life is – that doesn't mean a giving-in, but a recognition that my life includes controlled disease and has done for a long time. I also reckon that, if God is responsible for the cancer (which God must be as Creator), God is also responsible for the fact I am still alive – i.e. that people are intelligent enough to be developing weapons in the fight against cancer at a rate of knots these days. My drug (currently second-line treatment, being considered as first-line) wasn't in general use even as little as seven and a half years ago, when I was first diagnosed. In my Grandma's day (she died when Dad was four), I'd have been dead long since, with no second chances.

I am expecting to be given permission to retire early on health grounds (an enhanced pension provision on those grounds makes such a move financially viable). From a practical point of view I will be listed as a minister in a neighbouring circuit. I do have belief in God – I wouldn't have survived this long without a strong sense of accompaniment on the journey and I am happy to explore faith with other people, but I think life can be more than just a trial (as you observed!). I think it can be pretty shitty! And loads of people have it much worse than me. I don't understand why I have such a strong sense that it is possible to live in the Life Flow, and then you only have to watch the news to know that so many people don't ever get a chance to consider being part of that Life Flow, before they are blown away, humiliated or whatever by other people, war, drought, disease... Have I got you reaching for the gin yet?!

A twelve-hour working day – I'll think of you before my snooze! Jeremy is permanently 2-10pm – think I told you that. He is fit these days, as he cycles to work. He really is getting better again (I told you he'd had quite a struggle with depression?). I know, because he is busily planting seeds again, something he had stopped doing. He was referred for counselling when he finally admitted needing help sometime last autumn. He has been assessed and is waiting a place for one-to-one (can take up to a year to come to the top of the list). You know, the funny thing is, the paradox, is that he and I (individually, and as a couple) are probably happier currently than we have ever been! I can't quite work out why it takes life-threatening illness to make me a contented person! Something to do with realizing what does/doesn't matter in life maybe?! Or there again, just getting old and pickled in the brain!! Give our love to J.

Lesley.

EMAIL TO ALISON, JULY 2004

★

Dear Alison – My turn to take a while to reply. Trying to sort dates re holidays. Yes, if you have any time to come up on week beginning 9 August – we can fit in with you. Hopefully, we will have had a few days away ourselves the week before and may be able to get a late booking somewhere for the last week in August as well.

Treatment five last week. Brain struggling tonight. Ability to think dreadful. Coordination and energy disgusting. Still, nearly time for "Eastenders"! Saw doctor today for my last sick note (till end August). Last chemo hopefully 20 July. Clinically pleased with me – but it is a very unpleasant treatment. Still, we are surviving it!

I like the sun. Days like today are made more manageable when I can just get up and open all the doors and windows and sit in the sun in the backyard. When rain and grey are threatened (as tomorrow), that can be hard to keep spirits up when mobility and normal life patterns are grossly compromised. I can keep the house going, shop, cook and wash up (in my own time and at my own speed!). Realistically, not a lot else. My life has condensed immensely. But it is OK. Life goes on round about, which is good. I try to keep things 'normal' for everyone. Therefore, I don't think some people realise how ill I've been this time, but that is OK.

I need life to be normal and I feel it is an achievement that Jeremy can go to work without worrying about me, Katie can go to school and visit friends, Jamie can be in Paris as I write (celebrating the end of exams). I would be lost without the car. The dog keeps me exercised, but people do not always realise how much physically/mentally it costs to do the things I do. I am not complaining. Just writing some of the things I was thinking about lying on the bed this afternoon.

I have been lent the book you mentioned – I would like to see the article. But when I will be able to read it, I don't know. My ability to read is decreasing (poor concentration). Have several excellent books on the go, but have only managed to complete "The Godfather" since April. That was good. Got Mario Puzo's "The Family" on the go now. Can't always concentrate through a complete article in the local paper! Can manage "Eastenders" – they only talk in 'sound-bites'! Never doubted "the children" were a source of joy and delight to you and Adrian and that you are an excellent auntie and uncle. Bet you are looking forward to the end of term!!!!

Love Lesley X

EMAIL TO IAN, 15 JULY 2004

★

Dear Ian,

Didn't know you couldn't swim – did you never have lessons at school? Your relaxing Sunday sounded good. Baggy Cat is meowling behind me, as he gets as close to Jeremy as possible. He is our big black and white cat (once a rescue creature) and he needs quite a lot of affection. Sophie is sitting close to Jeremy on the other side, well as close as she can get given there is no room on the settee that side and Jeremy is trying to read the paper! Wherever one black and white creature is, there you will usually find the other (Sophie is also black and white). When I go to sleep on the bed in the afternoon, I have to strategically arrange myself between them, though when they think no one is looking and there is no human to snuggle up to, they have been found back to back on the settee for warmth!

My last treatment was Tuesday. Doctors pleased with me. Did I ever tell you that when I was discussing with one how long I've lived with this, he admitted that, "You've beaten the bookies!" We have managed to get a late booking of a cottage in a hamlet in North Wales, near the LLeyn Peninsular, where I've never been, but want to go, because of the R.S. Thomas connections. Looking forward to a break, which we all need. Jamie will housesit, Katie supposed to be bringing a friend. Later, we're trying for a late deal to the sun (last week in August). Hopefully Jamie will come to that too and Mum & Dad will house and animal sit. Can't fly earlier, because of my treatment and Jeremy's firm has let him split his fortnight, though he obviously has to be off the week the factory is completely shut down.

Jeremy has gone to sit at the table with book, biscuit and cup of tea. Pepe (grey cat) now about to sit on his book! "Cats make you take a rest from work by sitting on it," says one of my fridge magnets!

I am feeling much better in myself. Just having to get my head round what I live with, but that reshuffling in my head is usually a sign I feel better. When I feel lousy, I just have to get through the day!

Weather wet, but warm. Apparently the position of the Gulf Stream this year is not favourable to the good weather we had last year, but there have been a lot of nice days. I know, because I have the doors and windows open and sit in the yard a lot. Helps me to keep positive. It would have been hard to cope with this through winter, or if the days had been perpetually grey.

Got the rabbits out today. I try to, if the weather doesn't preclude it, though sometimes I can't manage it physically. Cottontail (young, long-haired, male rabbit) gets depressed if he doesn't get out, because he was brought up in a shop, I think. A very sociable little fella – Jeremy's favourite. Flopsy is mine – she is such a character. Mopsy is just one huge fluffy bunny, with an ever-increasing dewlap! Yet they all get treated and fed exactly the same! It always tickles me how the different little individuals (guinea pigs included) have their favourite foods. The guinea pigs LOVE broccoli stalks – absolute favourites! Flopsy would be a terror in Mr. MacGregor's garden (remember Beatrix Potter?!), because she loves dark green cabbage leaves. She is also very partial to the frilly bits on celery stalks. Mopsy's favourites are probably apples. Cottontail will eat those on the quiet, though I recently discovered that his favourite are the sweet little leaves in the centre of a cabbage. He doesn't always seem to eat much, though he runs round and round his cage in the yard, and sprays wee all over his territory (including Mopsy in the cage next door!). Hope you enjoyed that little diversionary tale about the animals – watching them is very good for my well being! As is walking Sophie!

Thinking of you.

Lesley X

EMAIL TO SUE, 31 AUGUST 2004

★

Dear Sue – We must have had the same week in Wales – 31st July onwards? Very hot, sunny beach weather on Lleyn Peninsular, staying at a cottage near Pwhelli. Lovely. Just come back from a week in Brittany. Mild and changeable weather there, but relaxing and enjoyable holiday. We have treated ourselves this year – thought we deserved it!

Treatment finished for now. Hair growing back. Gradually recovering my stamina. Now taking a new hormone drug (Exemestane), to try and maintain level of control of disease achieved by chemotherapy. See my specialist again in October – it will have been six weeks since I last saw him by then, so that makes a change from being constantly in and out of hospital!

Relieved to be retired, which I officially am from tomorrow (1 September) – no longer got the energy for paid employment, though I am enjoying being a full-time homemaker (never would have believed I'd say that twenty years ago!). Amazing how much kids need you around in the background even when they're getting big. Jamie is off to Nottingham Trent University in a couple of weeks, so we are preparing for that.

I have appreciated prayer support. Suppose my request for now would be that I continue to have the mental strength to live with this controlled disease. I am at a stage of acceptance that I never was when first diagnosed – i.e. that this is what I have to live with, but some days, it is a bit hard and nerve-wracking. It isn't going to go away, but today (i.e. at this moment) it is still in control. I am better at taking each day, each moment as it comes. But that's where prayer support comes in – so that I don't run away with the thoughts of what it might be like tomorrow, the day after or next year. That way madness lies! When diagnosed, I'm sure no-one would have expected me to get beyond the initial five years, not with simultaneous cancers that had both already gone into my lymph system. So, prayer alongside the excellent medical facilities available to me here has achieved something over the years!

Best regards to you and Pauline. I am so pleased with the way things are working out at B, and hope that the interviewing process will be successful.

From Lesley

EMAIL TO SUE, 3 SEPTEMBER 2004

★

I don't know that I would call it as positive an outcome as I'd hoped for – maybe that's what I mean about still needing prayers for living with my condition. Each treatment makes your reality clearer. You learn to cope, but though the treatment has been effective, its not necessarily worked as well as you would have hoped, or as effectively as past treatments might have done.

The main thing is that it is getting lonely, and I don't know if you will be able to understand that. Eight years since diagnosis. Anyone I know for whom it's been that long since diagnosis is either 'better' now and hopefully going to stay that way (past the 'magic' five years without recurrence), or they have died. One of my good friends, Sue, died last year. She lived for ten years with the disease controlled in her bones. She amazed the medics. I think of her a lot, because (retrospectively) I understand things she said and did, and she is still a strong mentor for me, though she is not physically still around. At the moment, I don't know on a close personal level other people who've lived with this as long as me. The situation will change as more and more people live with controlled disease. Apart from Sue, two of my other close, supportive friends also died last year.

And it's like lots of other life situations – if you haven't lived with it, some of the issues relating to it are not immediately obvious to understand. With Sue or Kath or Nell, I could have conversations that ranged from raucous laughter to comparing notes on how we lived and coped. Each of them knew when they had come to the end of their road and when medicine could do no more. I suppose I miss their companionship. The hospital has given me a support group number, but I don't feel I need a group as such. I don't particularly want to hear how other people feel about diagnosis or how their treatments work/don't work. I'm past all that. I would just like to chat to someone at a similar stage to me, trying to incorporate the reality of living with cancer into ordinary life. Will be thinking/praying round 7th for B.

Lesley

LETTER, 1 NOVEMBER 2004

★

Dear J – I have recently been forwarded a copy of your autumn letter, I don't know by whom. Having read it, I have considered carefully whether or not to write this letter, and have decided that I will, because you write in the public domain and have a particular ministry of spirituality that means your work affects the lives of other people.

There are some observations that I would like to make and will do so in "reply" to the points in your letter:

I am sorry that you have had breast cancer. I was first diagnosed with the disease in 1996 and have lived with it in a "controlled" way since then. It is not a nice disease and the treatments, though much improved from the past, are unpleasant.

I have discovered something of what I think you mean by "abundance" in the care of folk around me and the care beyond measure of an excellent nearby cancer centre. These both contribute to the continuation of my present life and to the fact that I am well at the moment.

I agree that "pretending piety" is not an option with God, but why should we assume that it be one in the first place? If God is Creator, God must take full responsibility for creation, including its xxxx-ups; cancer being one such, that I feel no need whatsoever to be polite to God about. I am however, immensely grateful for the creative skill of men and women, made in the likeness of God (as the book of "Genesis" in the Old Testament suggests), which enables intervention and treatment in situations of cancer, that can sometimes, somewhat remedy its effects and lead to a measure of healing taking place.

You wonder what would happen if you "told it as it was". I would like to suggest to you that, if you did so, some Church folk might not be so accommodating of your writing. The first time I wrote to "The Methodist Recorder" about my cancer, the article was highlighted in a local church. The second time, after a cancer recurrence, when life was harder to manage, "telling it how it was" went quietly unnoticed/ignored.

The road that involves living with cancer is not an easy one, and companionship with God on that route is sometimes hard to discern, and constantly being remade, reforged. Disease and its treatment take away our creativity, our concentration, and our spirituality. This is part of the way that it is – must we make excuses for God's apparent "absence" through it? That said, I ask myself, if my children, my husband, even my pets, were as afraid as I have been sometimes in the course of this illness, would I leave them to, "turn the corner of (their) fear, or leap the gap of unknowing on (their) own", as you suggest God has done to you? Then again, would I leave them to the "patience" of my "with-drawal" from them in such distress, and by such patronizing "patience" imply that the fault was somehow theirs for being so distressed in the first place (the implication being that, if only they understood what I was trying to teach them, they would not be afraid). If I wouldn't do such things to those I love, why on earth, or heaven, would God do them to me?

My husband and children are precisely the reason that I don't want to "die through this", though I have had to adjust over the years to the fact that such may be a likely outcome of this disability. Yet, I have come to feel quite strongly that, if I do die of my cancer, I will be held by God in that process, as I have always been held (though I admit, not always discernibly to me, except in the presence of the people round about me – who are the ones who so often provide God's hands and feet, ears and voice in the here and now). In the end, I suspect that the real anguish of death for me will be in the leave-taking that must occur from those I love.

J, I will never agree with you, and I do find the idea "offensive" (not "awesome", just plain "offensive") that this cancer is somehow a gift of God's "endless and eternal love for me." You are the second Christian woman writer I have read, who seems to want to view cancer as some kind of a gift from God. For myself, I partly judge a gift by how much I want to share it, and I would never give such a "gift" as cancer to anyone I love, nor even my worst enemy. I strongly refute the suggestion that cancer is any kind of a "gift" – I have never believed that in the eight years that this disease has been a companion to my life. Neither do I believe, that God has inflicted it on me. It seems to me that cancer is part of life, in all its fragility and brokenness. The gift of God lies in the ability to live with this condition creatively (wherein, I imagine, lies your "abundance") and in God's help, through friends, family and medics, to cope day by day.

I am glad that you feel yourself to be held in the abyss. I can accept your writing as your way of coping with what disease has done to your life. I do not accept it as a voice "also not mine", because that implies that the idea of cancer being a "gift" comes at God's suggestion. If that were so, I would not wish for a relationship with your God, or contemplation of the journey that implies towards understanding the likes of Auschwitz and beyond.

Creative process is mystery. Creative process impels me to write this letter – does it need to be sent, or do I just need to write it? You were frightened by your inability to write through your cancer treatment, what if you had been unable to write again ever? What if your cancer meant that your own particular ministry had been completely taken away from you?

I am no longer able to dialogue in terms of love, "that is not only for everyone but is also for us personally". Such an "unshakeable foundation" no longer defines my own understanding of God; though I too experience the energy released through creativity and the efficacy of "the small steps forward we take when everything appears to be against us."

You talk of "transformative energy". Hmm. How does that apply when the future no longer exists for the individual? When the transformation can only be into a deep unknown?

You write of sending your garden to your reader, "not as it is, but as it might be". If you could accept your garden as it is, rather than as it might be, I would offer to show you mine in its dereliction; for even there lie the seeds of hope for which you yearn. The seeds of hope are the gift. The cancer is not. Maybe the "storms" (and the darkness) are also the Life.

Yours, Lesley Whitehead.

EPILOGUE: 26 JANUARY 2005

★

The days are drawing out. The park gates close at 5pm now (instead of 4pm). Sophie and I have seen the first snowdrops on our daily squirrel-hunt. The hormone drug Exemestane (taken as a tiny tablet once a day) is doing a good job controlling my cancer and, so far, there has been no return of the lymphodema in my left arm. My consultant oncologist is pleased with my progress and I am only on three-monthly check-ups at the hospital (so nice not to have to go more often). Retirement is stimulating and enriching and my friend, Jose, is still alive. His first stay of execution came four hours before he was due to be killed on 10 July 2002. This month, he received a second stay, some days before his due date of death on 20 January. A return to Texas in retirement? We'll see!

BIBLIOGRAPHY

Article re death of Polly Havers. *Daily Express,* June 24 2004.

Atwood, Margaret (1979) *Surfacing.* London, Virago Press Ltd.

Baisley, Barbara (2000) *No Easy Answers: An Exploration Of Suffering.* Peterborough, Epworth Press.

Bon Jovi (1995) *These Days.* Polygram Records, Inc.

Clive's Cat's Cartoons. Available from: www.clivescats.com

Collins, A.S. (1946) *Treasury Of English Verse New And Old.* Foxton, near Cambridge, University Tutorial Press Ltd.

Cotter, Jim (1994) *Prayer At Night: A Book For The Darkness.* Sheffield, Cairns Publications.

Daly, Mary (1998) *Quintessence: Realizing the Archaic Future.* Boston, Massachusetts, Beacon Press.

Diamond, John (1999) *C: Because Cowards Get Cancer Too.* London, Vermillion.

Harding, Luke (2002) A Vision Of Hell In Indian City Gorging On Violence. *Guardian,* Saturday March 2 2002.

Hart, Josephine (1991) *Damage* London, Arrow Books Ltd.

Harvey, Anne *No One Left And No One Came: Adlestrop, By Edward Thomas.* London, BBC Radio Four (11.30am, June 28 2001).

Jones, Richard G. (Committee Chair) (1983) *Hymns & Psalms: A Methodist And Ecumenical Hymn Book.* London, Methodist Publishing House.

Keane, Fergal *Panorama: Mugabe – The Price Of Silence.* London, BBC2 (March 10 2002).

Keating, Ronan (2000) *Ronan.* Polydor Ltd. UK.

Keay, Kathy (1994) *Laughter, Silence & Shouting: An Anthology Of*

Women's Prayers. London, HarperCollins.

Keay, Kathy (1996) *Dancing On Mountains: An Anthology Of Women's Spiritual Writings*. London, HarperCollins.

Levi, Primo (1987) *If This Is A Man. The Truce*. Great Britain, Abacus.

Meatloaf (1993) *Bat Out Of Hell II: Back Into Hell*. Virgin Records Ltd.

Metzger, Bruce (For the Committee of Translators) (1989) *New Revised Standard Version Bible*. London, Collins Publishers.

Norris, Pamela (Editor) (1991) *Sound The Deep Waters: Women's Romantic Poetry In The Victorian Age*. London, Little, Brown & Company (Bullfinch Press).

Philip, Neil (Editor) (1990) *A Family Treasury Of Poetry*. Oxon, Dorling Kindersley.

Puzo, Mario (1998) *The Godfather*. London, Arrow Books.

Sarton, May (1978) *A Reckoning*. New York, W.W. Norton & Company Inc.

Shreve, Anita (1999) *The Pilot's Wife*. Great Britain, Abacus.

Springsteen, Bruce (1995) *Greatest Hits*. Sony Music Entertainment Inc.

Thomas, R.S. (1990) *Counterpoint*. Newcastle-Upon-Tyne, Bloodaxe Books Ltd.

Thomas, R.S. (1996) *No Truce With The Furies*. Newcastle-Upon-Tyne, Bloodaxe Books Ltd.

Traherne, Thomas (1988) *Centuries of Meditation*. Bridge Logos Publishing.

Travis (2001) *The Invisible Band*. Sony/ATV Music Publishing Ltd.

Vanstone, W.H. (1998) *Love's Endeavour, Love's Expense: The Response of Being To The Love Of God*. London, Darton, Longman & Todd.

Whitaker, Agnes (Editor) (1984) *All In The End Is Harvest: An Anthology For Those Who Grieve*. London, Darton, Longman

& Todd (in association with Cruse).

Wiesel, Elie (1981) Penguin Books Ltd., Middlesex, England. *Night*.

Wild Goose Worship Group (1999) *A Wee Worship Book*. Glasgow, Wild Goose Publications.

Wilkinson, Bruce (2001) *The Prayer Of Jabez*. U.S.A., Multnomah Publishers.